Virtual Clinical Excursions—Pediatrics

for

Wong's Essentials of Pediatric Nursing,
8th Edition

Virtual Clinical Excursions—Pediatrics

for

Wong's Essentials of Pediatric Nursing, 8th Edition

prepared by

David Wilson, RN, MS, RNC
Adjunct Faculty
Langston University
Tulsa, Oklahoma

Adjunct Faculty
Southern Nazarene University
Tulsa, Oklahoma

Staff, Children's Hospital Urgent Care Center
St. Francis Hospital
Tulsa, Oklahoma

Marilyn J. Hockenberry, PhD, RN-CS, PNP, FAAN
Director, Center for Clinical Research
Nurse Scientist, Texas Children's Hospital

Director of Nurse Practitioners
Texas Children's Cancer Center

Professor, Department of Pediatrics
Baylor College of Medicine
Houston, Texas

Patrick Barrera, BS
Research Program Coordinator
Center for Nursing Research
Texas Children's Hospital
Houston, Texas

software developed by

Wolfsong Informatics, LLC
Tucson, Arizona

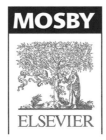

11830 Westline Industrial Dr.
St. Louis, Missouri 63146

VIRTUAL CLINICAL EXCURSIONS—PEDIATRICS FOR
WONG'S ESSENTIALS OF PEDIATRIC NURSING,
EIGHTH EDITION

Copyright © 2009 by Mosby, Inc., an affiliate of Elsevier Inc.

ISBN 978-0-323-05757-8

Notice

Knowledge and best practice in this field are constantly changing. As new research and experience broaden
our knowledge, changes in practice, treatment and drug therapy may become necessary or appropriate.
Readers are advised to check the most current information provided (i) on procedures featured or (ii) by the
manufacturer of each product to be administered, to verify the recommended dose or formula, the method
and duration of administration, and contraindications. It is the responsibility of the practitioner, relying on
their own experience and knowledge of the patient, to make diagnoses, to determine dosages and the best
treatment for each individual patient, and to take all appropriate safety precautions. To the fullest extent of
the law, neither the Publisher nor the Authors assumes any liability for any injury and/or damage to persons
or property arising out or related to any use of the material contained in this book.

ISBN 978-0-323-05757-8

Editor: *Jeff Downing*
Associate Developmental Editor: *Daniel Witzofsky*
Project Manager: *Tracey Schriefer*
Book Production Manager: *Gayle May*

Printed in the United States of America

Last digit is the print number: 9 8 7 6 5 4

Workbook
prepared by

David Wilson, MS, RNC
Adjunct Faculty
Langston University
Tulsa, Oklahoma

Adjunct Faculty
Southern Nazarene University
Tulsa, Oklahoma

Staff, Children's Hospital Urgent Care Center
St. Francis Hospital
Tulsa, Oklahoma

Marilyn J. Hockenberry, PhD, RN-CS, PNP, FAAN
Director, Center for Clinical Research
Nurse Scientist, Texas Children's Hospital

Director of Nurse Practitioners
Texas Children's Cancer Center

Professor, Department of Pediatrics
Baylor College of Medicine
Houston, Texas

Contributing Editor

Patrick Barrera, BS
Research Program Coordinator
Center for Nursing Research
Texas Children's Hospital
Houston, Texas

Textbook

Marilyn J. Hockenberry, PhD, RN-CS, PNP, FAAN
Director, Center for Clinical Research
Nurse Scientist, Texas Children's Hospital

Director of Nurse Practitioners
Texas Children's Cancer Center

Professor, Department of Pediatrics
Baylor College of Medicine
Houston, Texas

David Wilson, MS, RNC
Adjunct Faculty
Langston University
Tulsa, Oklahoma

Adjunct Faculty
Southern Nazarene University
Tulsa, Oklahoma

Staff, Children's Hospital Urgent Care Center
St. Francis Hospital
Tulsa, Oklahoma

Reviewers

Chris L. Algren, EdD, MSN, RN
Professor and Associate Dean
Gordon E. Inman College of Health Sciences & Nursing
Belmont University
Nashville, Tennessee

Brenda Pavill, RN, FNP, PhD
Associate Professor
Department of Nursing
Misericordia University
Dallas, Pennsylvania

Contents

Table of Contents
Wong's Essentials of Pediatric Nursing, 8th Edition

Getting Started

GETTING SET UP

■ MINIMUM SYSTEM REQUIREMENTS

WINDOWS®

Windows Vista®, XP, 2000 (Recommend Windows XP/2000)
Pentium® III processor (or equivalent) @ 600 MHz (Recommend 800 MHz or better)
256 MB of RAM (Recommend 1 GB or more for Windows Vista)
800 x 600 screen size (Recommend 1024 x 768)
Thousands of colors
12x CD-ROM drive
Stereo speakers or headphones

Note: Windows Vista and XP require administrator privileges for installation.

MACINTOSH®

MAC OS X (up to 10.6.1)
Apple Power PC G3 @ 500 MHz or better
128 MB of RAM (Recommend 256 MB or more)
800 x 600 screen size (Recommend 1024 x 768)
Thousands of colors
12x CD-ROM drive
Stereo speakers or headphones

■ INSTALLATION INSTRUCTIONS

WINDOWS

1. Insert the *Virtual Clinical Excursions—Pediatrics* CD-ROM.
2. The setup screen should appear automatically if the current product is not already installed. Windows Vista users may be asked to authorize additional security prompts.
3. Follow the onscreen instructions during the setup process.

   If the setup screen does *not* appear automatically (and *Virtual Clinical Excursions— Pediatrics* has not been installed already):
   a. Click the **My Computer** icon on your desktop or on your Start menu.
   b. Double-click on your CD-ROM drive.
   c. If installation does not start at this point:
      (1) Click the **Start** icon on the taskbar and select the **Run** option.
      (2) Type d:\setup.exe (where "d:\" is your CD-ROM drive) and press **OK**.
      (3) Follow the onscreen instructions for installation.

MACINTOSH

1. Insert the *Virtual Clinical Excursions—Pediatrics* CD in the CD-ROM drive. The disk icon will appear on your desktop.

2. Double-click on the disk icon.

3. Double-click on the VCEPE_MAC run file.

Note: Virtual Clinical Excursions—Pediatrics for Macintosh does not have an installation setup and can only be run directly from the CD.

■ HOW TO USE VIRTUAL CLINICAL EXCURSIONS—PEDIATRICS

WINDOWS

1. Double-click on the *Virtual Clinical Excursions—Pediatrics* icon located on your desktop.
2. Or navigate to the program via the Windows Start menu.

Note: If your computer uses Windows Vista, right-click on the desktop shortcut and choose **Properties**. In the Compatability Mode, check the box for "Run as Administrator." Below is a screen capture to show what this looks like.

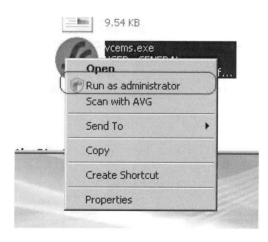

MACINTOSH

1. Insert the *Virtual Clinical Excursions—Pediatrics* CD in the CD-ROM drive. The disk icon will appear on your desktop.

2. Double-click on the disk icon.

3. Double-click on the VCEPE_MAC run file.

■ SCREEN SETTINGS

For best results, your computer monitor resolution should be set at a minimum of 800 x 600. The number of colors displayed should be set to "thousands or higher" (High Color or 16 bit) or "millions of colors" (True Color or 24 bit).

Windows

1. From the **Start** menu, select **Control Panel** (on some systems, you will first go to **Settings**, then to **Control Panel**).
2. Double-click on the **Display** icon.
3. Click on the **Settings** tab.
4. Under **Screen resolution** use the slider bar to select **800 by 600 pixels**.
5. Access the **Colors** drop-down menu by clicking on the down arrow.
6. Select **High Color (16 bit)** or **True Color (24 bit)**.
7. Click on **OK**.
8. You may be asked to verify the setting changes. Click **Yes**.
9. You may be asked to restart your computer to accept the changes. Click **Yes**.

Macintosh

1. Select the **Monitors** control panel.
2. Select **800 x 600** (or similar) from the **Resolution** area.
3. Select **Thousands** or **Millions** from the **Color Depth** area.

■ WEB BROWSERS

Supported web browsers include Microsoft Internet Explorer (IE) version 7.0 or higher and Mozilla 3.0 or higher.

If you use America Online® (AOL) for web access, you will need AOL version 4.0 or higher and one of the browsers listed above. Do not use earlier versions of AOL with earlier versions of IE, because you will have difficulty accessing many features.

For best results with AOL:
- Connect to the Internet using AOL version 4.0 or higher.
- Open a private chat within AOL (this allows the AOL client to remain open, without asking whether you wish to disconnect while minimized).
- Minimize AOL.
- Launch a recommended browser.

■ TECHNICAL SUPPORT

Technical support for this product is available 24 hours a day, seven days a week, excluding holidays. Before calling, be sure that your computer meets the minimum system requirements to run this software. Inside the United States and Canada, call 1-800-222-9570. Outside North America, call 314-447-8094. You may also fax your questions to 314-447-8078 or contact Technical Support through e-mail: technical.support@elsevier.com.

Trademarks: Windows, Macintosh, Pentium, and America Online are registered trademarks.

Copyright © 2009 by Mosby, Inc., an affiliate of Elsevier Inc.

All rights reserved. No part of this product may be reproduced or transmitted in any form or by any means, electronic or mechanical, including input or storage in any information system, without written permission from the publisher.

ACCESSING *Virtual Clinical Excursions—Pediatrics* FROM EVOLVE

The product you have purchased is part of the Evolve family of online courses and learning resources. Please read the following information thoroughly to get started.

To access your instructor's course on Evolve:

Your instructor will provide you with the username and password needed to access this specific course on the Evolve Learning System. Once you have received this information, please follow these instructions:

1. Go to the Evolve student page (http://evolve.elsevier.com/student).

2. Enter your username and password in the **Login to My Evolve** area and click the **Login** button.

3. You will be taken to your personalized **My Evolve** page, where the course will be listed in the **My Courses** module.

TECHNICAL REQUIREMENTS

To use an Evolve course, you will need access to a computer that is connected to the Internet and equipped with web browser software that supports frames. For optimal performance, it is recommended that you have speakers and use a high-speed Internet connection. However, slower dial-up modems (56 K minimum) are acceptable.

Whichever browser you use, the browser preferences must be set to enable cookies and the cache must be set to reload every time.

<u>**Enable Cookies**</u>

Browser	Steps
Internet Explorer (IE) 7.0 or higher	1. Select **Tools → Internet Options**. 2. Select **Privacy** tab. 3. Use the slider (slide down) to **Accept All Cookies**. 4. Click **OK**. -OR- 3. Click the **Advanced** button. 4. Click the check box next to **Override Automatic Cookie Handling**. 5. Click the **Accept** radio buttons under **First-party Cookies** and **Third-party Cookies**. 6. Click **OK**.
Mozilla Firefox 3.0 or higher	1. Select **Tools → Options**. 2. Select the **Privacy** icon. 3. Click to expand Cookies. 4. Select **Allow sites to set cookies**. 5. Click **OK**.

<u>**Set Cache to Always Reload a Page**</u>

Browser	Steps
Internet Explorer (IE) 7.0 or higher	1. Select **Tools → Internet Options**. 2. Select **General** tab. 3. Go to the **Temporary Internet Files** and click the **Settings** button. 4. Select the radio button for **Every visit to the page** and click **OK** when complete.
Mozilla Firefox 3.0 or higher	1. Select **Tools → Options**. 2. Select the **Privacy** icon. 3. Click to expand Cache. 4. Set the value to "0" in the **Use up to: __ MB of disk space for the cache** field. 5. Click **OK**.

Plug-Ins

 Adobe Acrobat Reader—With the free Acrobat Reader software, you can view and print Adobe PDF files. Many Evolve products offer student and instructor manuals, checklists, and more in this format!

Download at: http://www.adobe.com

 Apple QuickTime—Install this to hear word pronunciations, heart and lung sounds, and many other helpful audio clips within Evolve Online Courses!

Download at: http://www.apple.com

 Adobe Flash Player—This player will enhance your viewing of many Evolve web pages, as well as educational short-form to long-form animation within the Evolve Learning System!

Download at: http://www.adobe.com

 Adobe Shockwave Player—Shockwave is best for viewing the many interactive learning activities within Evolve Online Courses!

Download at: http://www.adobe.com

 Microsoft Word Viewer—With this viewer, Microsoft Word users can share documents with those who don't have Word, and users without Word can open and view Word documents. Many Evolve products have testbank, student and instructor manuals, and other documents available for downloading and viewing on your own computer!

Download at: http://www.microsoft.com

 Microsoft PowerPoint Viewer—With this viewer, you can access PowerPoint 97, 2000, and 2002 presentations even if you don't have PowerPoint. Many Evolve products have slides available for downloading and viewing on your own computer!

Download at: http://www.microsoft.com

SUPPORT INFORMATION

Live phone support is available to customers is available 24 hours a day, seven days a week, excluding holidays, to customers in the United States and Canada at **800-222-9570**. Support is also available through email at technical.support@elsevier.com.

Online 24/7 support can be accessed on the Evolve website (http://evolve.elsevier.com). Resources include:

- Guided tours
- Tutorials
- Frequently asked questions (FAQs)
- Online copies of course user guides
- And much more!

A QUICK TOUR

Welcome to *Virtual Clinical Excursions—Pediatrics*, a virtual hospital setting in which you can work with multiple complex patient simulations and also learn to access and evaluate the information resources that are essential for high-quality patient care. The virtual hospital, Pacific View Regional Hospital, has realistic architecture and access to patient rooms, a Nurses' Station, and a Medication Room.

■ BEFORE YOU START

Make sure you have your textbook nearby when you use the *Virtual Clinical Excursions— Pediatrics* CD. You will want to consult topic areas in your textbook frequently while working with the CD and using this workbook.

■ HOW TO SIGN IN

- Enter your name on the Student Nurse identification badge.
- Now choose one of the four periods of care in which to work. In Periods of Care 1 through 3, you can actively engage in patient assessment, entry of data in the electronic patient record (EPR), and medication administration. Period of Care 4 presents the day in review. Highlight and click the appropriate period of care. (For this quick tour, choose **Period of Care 1: 0730-0815**.)
- This takes you to the Patient List screen (see example on page 11). Only the patients on the Pediatrics Floor are available. Note that the virtual time is provided in the box at the lower left corner of the screen (0731, since we chose Period of Care 1).

Note: If you choose to work during Period of Care 4: 1900-2000, the Patient List screen is skipped since you are not able to visit patients or administer medications during the shift. Instead, you are taken directly to the Nurses' Station, where the records of all the patients on the floor are available for your review.

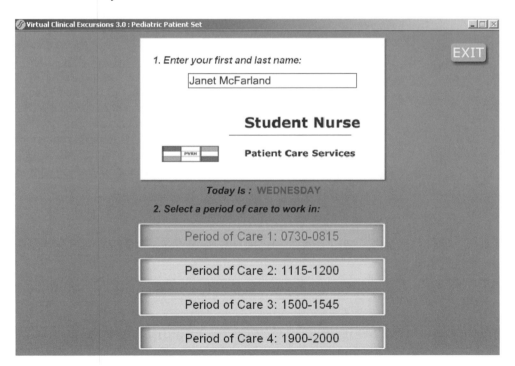

■ PATIENT LIST

PEDIATRICS UNIT

George Gonzalez (Room 301)
Diabetic ketoacidosis—An 11-year-old Hispanic male admitted for stabilization of blood glucose level and diabetic re-education associated with his diagnosis of type 1 diabetes mellitus. This patient's poor compliance with insulin therapy and dietary regime have resulted in frequent and repeated hospital admissions for DKA.

Tommy Douglas (Room 302)
Traumatic brain injury—A 6-year-old Caucasian male transferred from the Pediatric Intensive Care Unit in preparation for organ donation. This patient is status post ventriculostomy with negative intracerebral blood flow and requires extensive hemodynamic monitoring and support, along with compassionate family care.

Carrie Richards (Room 303)
Bronchiolitis—A 3½-month-old African-American female admitted with respiratory distress due to respiratory syncytial virus, along with dehydration and a poor nutritional status. Parent education and support are among her primary needs.

Stephanie Brown (Room 304)
Meningitis—A 3-year-old African-American female with a history of spastic cerebral palsy admitted for intravenous antibiotic therapy, neurologic monitoring, and support for a diagnosis of acute meningitis. Maintenance of physical and occupational programs addressing her mobility limitations complicate her acute care stay.

Tiffany Sheldon (Room 305)
Anorexia nervosa—A 14-year-old Caucasian female admitted for dehydration, electrolyte imbalance, and malnutrition following a syncope episode at home. This patient has a history of eating disorders, which have resulted in multiple hospital admissions and strained family dynamics between mother and daughter.

■ HOW TO SELECT A PATIENT

- You can choose one or more patients to work with from the Patient List by checking the box to the left of the patient name(s). For this quick tour, select Stephanie Brown. (In order to receive a scorecard for a patient, the patient must be selected before proceeding to the Nurses' Station.)
- Click on **Get Report** to the right of the medical records number (MRN) to view a summary of the patient's care during the 12-hour period before your arrival on the unit.
- After reviewing the report, click on **Go to Nurses' Station** in the right lower corner to begin your care. (*Note:* If you have been assigned to care for multiple patients, you can click on **Return to Patient List** to select and review the report for each additional patient before going to the Nurses' Station.)

Note: Even though the Patient List is initially skipped when you sign in to work for Period of Care 4, you can still access this screen if you wish to review the shift report for any of the patients. To do so, simply click on **Patient List** near the top left corner of the Nurses' Station (or click on the clipboard to the left of the Kardex). Then click on **Get Report** for the patient(s) whose care you are reviewing. This may be done during any period of care.

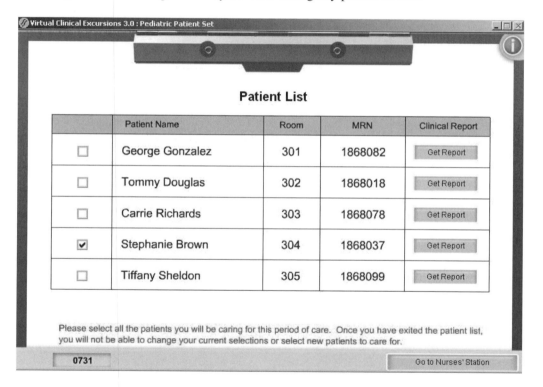

■ HOW TO FIND A PATIENT'S RECORDS

NURSES' STATION

Within the Nurses' Station, you will see:

1. A clipboard that contains the patient list for that floor.
2. A chart rack with patient charts labeled by room number, a notebook labeled Kardex, and a notebook labeled MAR (Medication Administration Record).
3. A desktop computer with access to the Electronic Patient Record (EPR).
4. A tool bar across the top of the screen that can also be used to access the Patient List, EPR, Chart, MAR, and Kardex. This tool bar is also accessible from each patient's room.
5. A Drug Guide containing information about the medications you are able to administer to your patients.
6. A tool bar across the bottom of the screen that can be used to access the Floor Map, patient rooms, Medication Room, and Drug Guide.

As you run your cursor over an item, it will be highlighted. To select, simply double-click on the item. As you use these resources, you will always be able to return to the Nurses' Station by clicking on the **Return to Nurses' Station** bar located in the right lower corner of your screen.

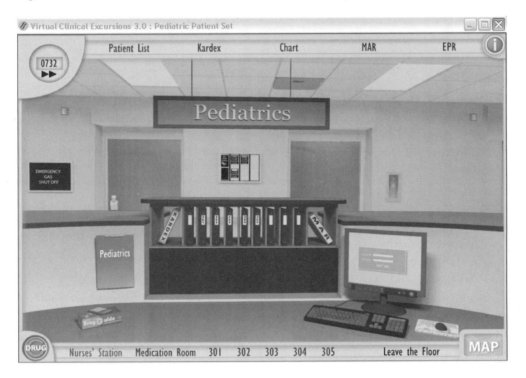

MEDICATION ADMINISTRATION RECORD (MAR)

The MAR icon located on the tool bar at the top of your screen accesses current 24-hour medications for each patient. Click on the icon and the MAR will open. (*Note:* You can also access the MAR by clicking on the MAR notebook on the far right side of the book rack in the center of the screen.) Within the MAR, tabs on the right side of the screen allow you to select patients by room number. Be careful to make sure you select the correct tab number for *your* patient rather than simply reading the first record that appears after the MAR opens. Each MAR sheet lists the following:

- Medications
- Route and dosage of each medication
- Times of administration of each medication

Note: The MAR changes each day. Expired MARs are stored in the patients' charts.

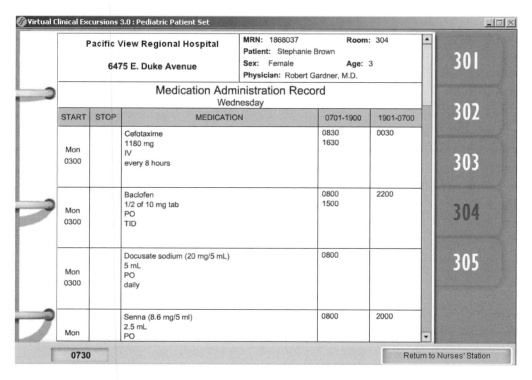

CHARTS

To access patient charts, either click on the **Chart** icon at the top of your screen or anywhere within the chart rack in the center of the Nurses' Station screen. When the close-up view appears, the individual charts are labeled by room number. To open a chart, click on the room number of the patient whose chart you wish to review. The patient's name and allergies will appear on the left side of the screen, along with a list of tabs on the right side of the screen, allowing you to view the following data:

- Allergies
- Physician's Orders
- Physician's Notes
- Nurse's Notes
- Laboratory Reports
- Diagnostic Reports
- Surgical Reports
- Consultations
- Patient Education
- History and Physical
- Nursing Admission
- Expired MARs
- Consents
- Mental Health
- Admissions
- Emergency Department

Information appears in real time. The entries are in reverse chronologic order, so use the down arrow at the right side of each chart page to scroll down to view previous entries. Flip from tab to tab to view multiple data fields or click on **Return to Nurses' Station** in the lower right corner of the screen to exit the chart.

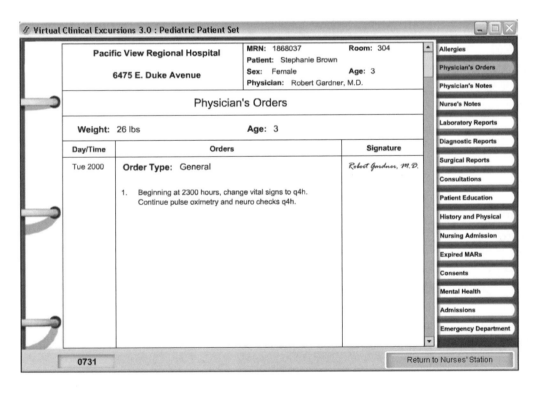

ELECTRONIC PATIENT RECORD (EPR)

The EPR can be accessed from the computer in the Nurses' Station or from the EPR icon located in the tool bar at the top of your screen. To access a patient's EPR:

- Click on either the computer screen or the **EPR** icon.
- Your username and password are automatically filled in.
- Click on **Login** to enter the EPR.
- *Note:* Like the MAR, the EPR is arranged numerically. Thus when you enter, you are initially shown the records of the patient in the lowest room number on the floor. To view the correct data for *your* patient, remember to select the correct room number, using the drop-down menu for the Patient field at the top left corner of the screen.

The EPR used in Pacific View Regional Hospital represents a composite of commercial versions being used in hospitals. You can access the EPR:

- to review existing data for a patient (by room number).
- to enter data you collect while working with a patient.

The EPR is updated daily, so no matter what day or part of a shift you are working, there will be a current EPR with the patient's data from the past days of the current hospital stay. This type of simulated EPR allows you to examine how data for different attributes have changed over time, as well as to examine data for all of a patient's attributes at a particular time. The EPR is fully functional (as it is in a real-life hospital). You can enter such data as blood pressure, breath sounds, and certain treatments. The EPR will not, however, allow you to enter data for a previous time period. Use the arrows at the bottom of the screen to move forward and backward in time.

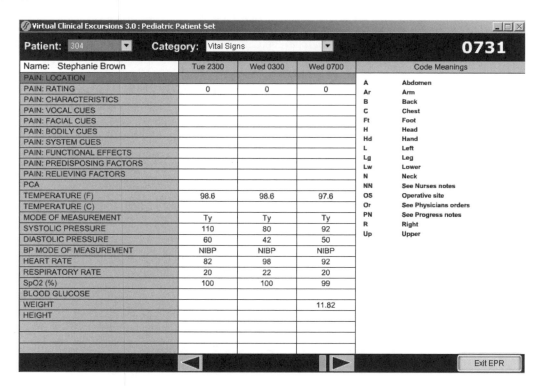

Virtual Clinical Excursions 3.0 : Pediatric Patient Set

Patient: 304   Category: Vital Signs   0731

Name: Stephanie Brown	Tue 2300	Wed 0300	Wed 0700	Code Meanings	
PAIN: LOCATION				A	Abdomen
PAIN: RATING	0	0	0	Ar	Arm
PAIN: CHARACTERISTICS				B	Back
PAIN: VOCAL CUES				C	Chest
PAIN: FACIAL CUES				Ft	Foot
PAIN: BODILY CUES				H	Head
PAIN: SYSTEM CUES				Hd	Hand
PAIN: FUNCTIONAL EFFECTS				L	Left
PAIN: PREDISPOSING FACTORS				Lg	Leg
PAIN: RELIEVING FACTORS				Lw	Lower
PCA				N	Neck
TEMPERATURE (F)	98.6	98.6	97.6	NN	See Nurses notes
TEMPERATURE (C)				OS	Operative site
MODE OF MEASUREMENT	Ty	Ty	Ty	Or	See Physicians orders
SYSTOLIC PRESSURE	110	80	92	PN	See Progress notes
DIASTOLIC PRESSURE	60	42	50	R	Right
BP MODE OF MEASUREMENT	NIBP	NIBP	NIBP	Up	Upper
HEART RATE	82	98	92		
RESPIRATORY RATE	20	22	20		
SpO2 (%)	100	100	99		
BLOOD GLUCOSE					
WEIGHT			11.82		
HEIGHT					

Exit EPR

At the top of the EPR screen, you can choose patients by their room numbers. In addition, you have access to 17 different categories of patient data. To change patients or data categories, click the down arrow to the right of the room number or category.

The categories of patient data in the EPR as as follows:

- Vital Signs
- Respiratory
- Cardiovascular
- Neurologic
- Gastrointestinal
- Excretory
- Musculoskeletal
- Integumentary
- Reproductive
- Psychosocial
- Wounds and Drains
- Activity
- Hygiene and Comfort
- Safety
- Nutrition
- IV
- Intake and Output

Remember, each hospital selects its own codes. The codes used in the EPR at Pacific View Regional Hospital may be different from ones you have seen in your clinical rotations. Take some time to acquaint yourself with the codes. Within the Vital Signs category, click on any item in the left column (e.g., Pain: Characteristics). In the far-right column, you will see a list of code meanings for the possible findings and/or descriptors for that assessment area.

You will use the codes to record the data you collect as you work with patients. Click on the box in the last time column to the right of any item and wait for the code meanings applicable to that entry to appear. Select the appropriate code to describe your assessment findings and type it in the box. (*Note:* If no cursor appears within the box, click on the box again until the blue shading disappears and the blinking cursor appears.) Once the data are typed in this box, they are entered into the patient's record for this period of care only.

To leave the EPR, click on **Exit EPR** in the bottom right corner of the screen.

■ VISITING A PATIENT

From the Nurses' Station, click on the room number of the patient you wish to visit (in the tool bar at the bottom of your screen). Once you are inside the room, you will see a still photo of your patient in the top left corner. To verify that this is the correct patient, click on the **Check Armband** icon to the right of the photo. The patient's identification data will appear. If you click on **Check Allergies** (the next icon to the right), a list of the patient's allergies (if any) will replace the photo.

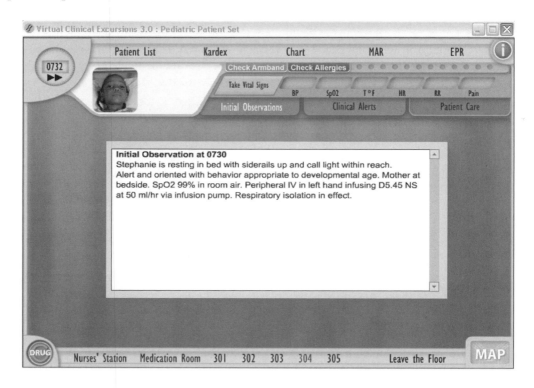

Also located in the patient's room are multiple icons you can use to assess the patient or the patient's medications. A virtual clock is provided in the upper left corner of the room to monitor your progress in real time. (*Note:* The fast-forward icon within the virtual clock will advance the time by 2-minute intervals when clicked.)

- The tool bar across the top of the screen allows you to check the **Patient List**, access the **EPR** to check or enter data, and view the patient's **Chart**, **MAR**, or **Kardex**.

- The **Take Vital Signs** icon allows you to measure the patient's up-to-the-minute blood pressure, oxygen saturation, temperature, heart rate, respiratory rate, and pain level.

- Each time you enter a patient's room, you are given an Initial Observation report to review (in the text box under the patient's photo). These notes are provided to give you a "look" at the patient as if you had just stepped into the room. You can also click on the **Initial Observations** icon to return to this box from other views within the patient's room. To the right of this icon is **Clinical Alerts**, a resource that allows you to make decisions about priority medication interventions based on emerging data collected in real time. Check this screen throughout your period of care to avoid missing critical information related to recently ordered or STAT medications.

- Clicking on **Patient Care** opens up three specific learning environments within the patient room: **Physical Assessment**, **Nurse-Client Interactions**, and **Medication Administration**.

- To perform a **Physical Assessment**, choose a body area (such as **Head & Neck**) from the column of yellow buttons. This activates a list of system subcategories for that body area (e.g., see **Sensory**, **Neurologic**, etc. in the green boxes). After you select the system you wish to evaluate, a brief description of the assessment findings will appear in a box to the right. A still photo provides a "snapshot" of how an assessment of this area might be done or what the finding might look like. For every body area, you can also click on **Equipment** on the right side of the screen.

- To the right of the Physical Assessment icon is **Nurse-Client Interactions**. Clicking on this icon will reveal the times and titles of any videos available for viewing. (*Note:* If the video you wish to see is not listed, this means you have not yet reached the correct virtual time to view that video. Check the virtual clock; you may return to access the video once its designated time has occurred—as long as you do so within the same period of care. Or you can click on the fast-forward icon within the virtual clock to advance the time by 2-minute intervals. You will then need to click again on **Patient Care** and **Nurse-Client Interactions** to refresh the screen.) To view a listed video, click on the white arrow to the right of the video title. Use the control buttons below the video to start, stop, pause, rewind, or fast-forward the action or to mute the sound.

- **Medication Administration** is the pathway that allows you to review and administer medications to a patient after you have prepared them in the Medication Room. This process is addressed further in the *How to Prepare Medications* section (pages 19-20) and in *Medications* (pages 26-30). For additional hands-on practice, see *Reducing Medication Errors* (pages 37-41).

■ HOW TO QUIT, CHANGE PATIENTS, OR CHANGE PERIODS OF CARE

How to Quit: From most screens, you may click the **Leave the Floor** icon on the bottom tool bar to the right of the patient room numbers. (*Note:* From some screens, you will first need to click an **Exit** button or **Return to Nurses' Station** before clicking **Leave the Floor**.) When the Floor Menu appears, click **Exit** to leave the program.

How to Change Patients or Periods of Care: To change patients, simply click on the new patient's room number. (You cannot receive a scorecard for a new patient, however, unless you have already selected that patient on the Patient List screen.) To change to a new period of care or to restart the virtual clock, click on **Leave the Floor** and then on **Restart the Program**.

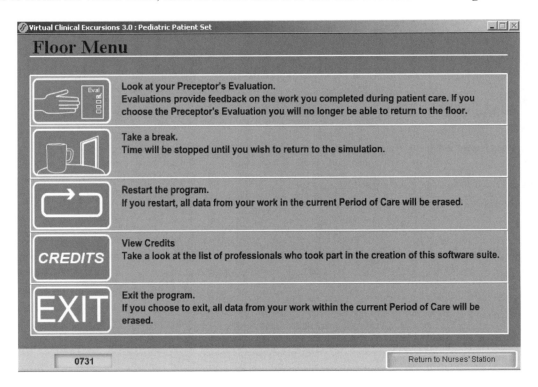

■ HOW TO PREPARE MEDICATIONS

From the Nurses' Station or the patient's room, you can access the Medication Room by clicking on the icon in the tool bar at the bottom of your screen to the left of the patient room numbers.

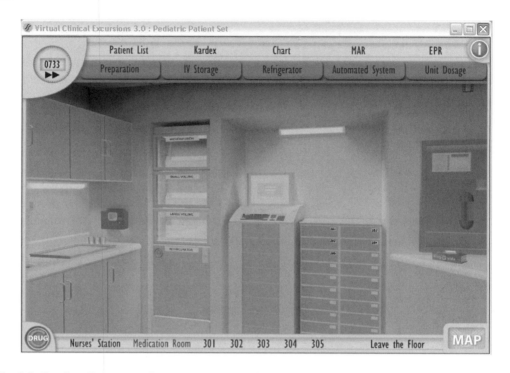

In the Medication Room you have access to the following (from left to right):

- A preparation area is located on the counter under the cabinets. To begin the medication preparation process, click on the tray on the counter or click on the **Preparation** icon at the top of the screen. The next screen leads you through a specific sequence (called the Preparation Wizard) to prepare medications one at a time for administration to a patient. However, no medication has been selected at this time. We will do this while working with a patient in *A Detailed Tour*. To exit this screen, click on **View Medication Room**.

- To the right of the cabinets (and above the refrigerator), IV storage bins are provided. Click on the bins themselves or on the **IV Storage** icon at the top of the screen. The bins are labeled **Microinfusion**, **Small Volume**, and **Large Volume**. Click on an individual bin to see a list of its contents. If you needed to prepare an IV medication at this time, you could click on the medication and its label would appear to the right under the patient's name. (*Note:* You can **Open** and **Close** any medication label by clicking the appropriate icon.) Next, you would click **Put Medication on Tray**. If you ever change your mind or decide that you have put the incorrect medication on the tray. you can reverse your actions by highlighting the medication on the tray and then clicking **Put Medication in Bin**. Click **Close Bin** in the right bottom corner to exit. **View Medication Room** brings you back to a full view of the entire room.

- A refrigerator is located under the IV storage bins to hold any medications that must be stored below room temperature. Click on the refrigerator door or on the **Refrigerator** icon at the top of the screen. Then click on the close-up view of the door to access the medications. When you are finished, click **Close Door** and then **View Medication Room**.

- To prepare controlled substances, click the **Automated System** icon at the top of the screen or click the computer monitor located to the right of the IV storage bins. A login screen will appear; your name and password are automatically filled in. Click **Login**. Select the patient for whom you wish to access medications; then select the correct medication drawer to open (they are stored alphabetically). Click **Open Drawer**, highlight the proper medication, and choose **Put Medication on Tray**. When you are finished, click **Close Drawer** and then **View Medication Room**.

- Next to the Automated System is a set of drawers identified by patient room number. To access these, click on the drawers or on the **Unit Dosage** icon at the top of the screen. This provides a close-up view of the drawers. To open a drawer, click on the room number of the patient you are working with. Next, click on the medication you would like to prepare for the patient, and a label will appear to the right, listing the medication strength, units, and dosage per unit. To exit, click **Close Drawer**; then click **View Medication Room**.

At any time, you can learn about a medication you wish to prepare for a patient by clicking on the **Drug** icon in the bottom left corner of the medication room screen or by clicking the **Drug Guide** book on the counter to the right of the unit dosage drawers. The **Drug Guide** provides information about the medications commonly included in nursing drug handbooks. Nutritional supplements and maintenance intravenous fluid preparations are not included. Highlight a medication in the alphabetical list; relevant information about the drug will appear in the screen below. To exit, click **Return to Medication Room**.

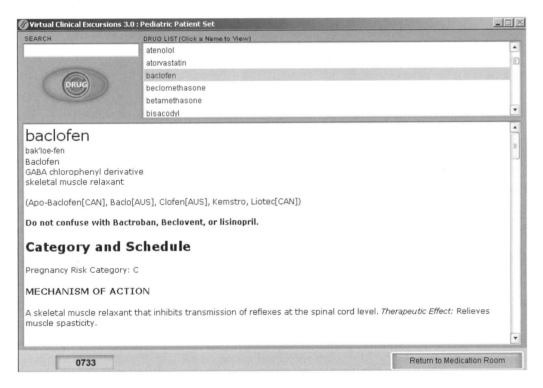

To access the MAR to review the medications ordered for a patient, click on the **MAR** icon located in the tool bar at the top of your screen and then click on the correct tab for your patient's room number. You may also click the **Review MAR** icon in the tool bar at the bottom of your screen from inside each medication storage area.

After you have chosen and prepared medications, go to the patient's room to administer them by clicking on the room number in the bottom tool bar. Inside the patient's room, click **Patient Care** and then **Medication Administration** and follow the proper administration sequence.

■ PRECEPTOR'S EVALUATIONS

When you have finished a session, click on **Leave the Floor** to go to the Floor Menu. At this point, you can click on the top icon (**Look at Your Preceptor's Evaluation**) to receive a score-card that provides feedback on the work you completed during patient care.

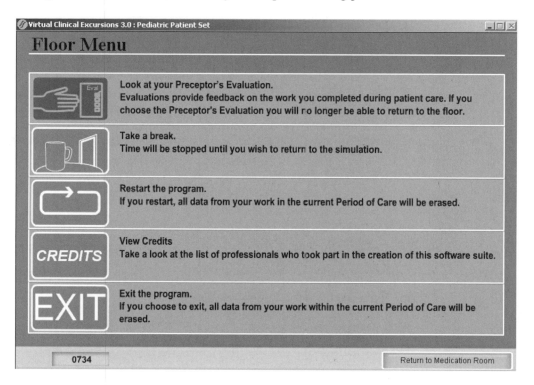

Evaluations are available for each patient you selected when you signed in for the current period of care. Click on the **Medication Scorecard** icon to see an example.

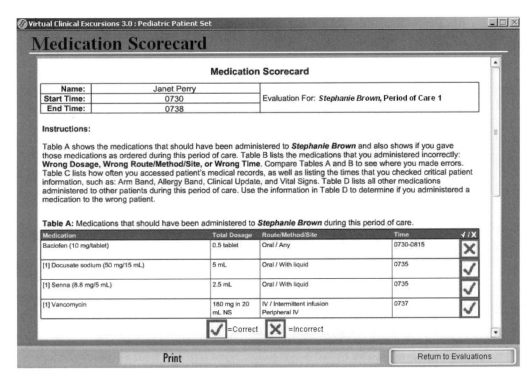

The scorecard compares the medications you administered to a patient during a period of care with what should have been administered. Table A lists the correct medications. Table B lists any medications that were administered incorrectly.

Remember, not every medication listed on the MAR should necessarily be given. For example, a patient might have an allergy to a drug that was ordered, or a medication might have been improperly transcribed to the MAR. Predetermined medication "errors" embedded within the program challenge you to exercise critical thinking skills and professional judgment when deciding to administer a medication, just as you would in a real hospital. Use all your available resources, such as the patient's chart and the MAR, to make your decision.

Table C lists the resources that were available to assist you in medication administration. It also documents whether and when you accessed these resources. For example, did you check the patient armband or perform a check of vital signs? If so, when?

You can click **Print** to get a copy of this report if needed. When you have finished reviewing the scorecard, click **Return to Evaluations** and then **Return to Menu**.

■ FLOOR MAP

To get a general sense of your location within the hospital, you can click on the **Map** icon found in the lower right corner of most of the screens in the *Virtual Clinical Excursions—Pediatrics* program. (*Note:* If you are following this quick tour step by step, you will need to **Restart the Program** from the Floor Menu, sign in again, and go to the Nurses' Station to access the map.) When you click the **Map** icon, a floor map appears, showing the layout of the floor you are currently on, as well as a directory of the patients and services on that floor. As you move your cursor over the directory list, the location of each room is highlighted on the map (and vice versa). The floor map can be accessed from the Nurses' Station, Medication Room, and each patient's room.

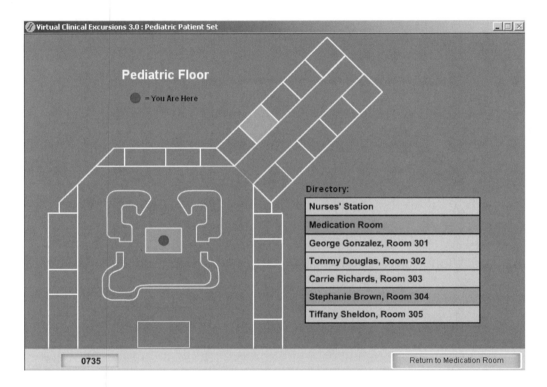

A DETAILED TOUR

If you wish to more thoroughly understand the capabilities of *Virtual Clinical Excursions—Pediatrics*, take a detailed tour by completing the following section. During this tour, we will work with a specific patient to introduce you to all the different components and learning opportunities available within the software.

■ WORKING WITH A PATIENT

Sign in for Period of Care 1 (0730-0815). From the Patient List, select Stephanie Brown in Room 304; however, do not go to the Nurses' Station yet.

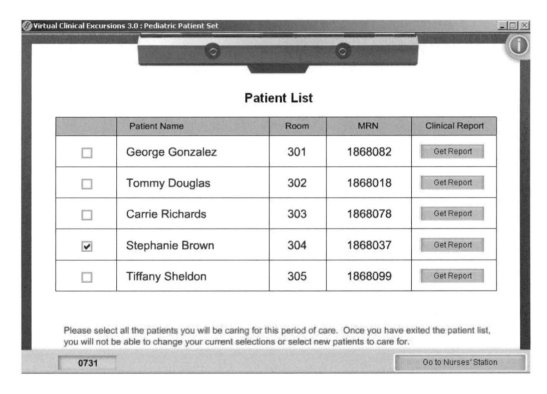

■ REPORT

In hospitals, when one shift ends and another begins, the outgoing nurse who attended a patient will give a verbal and sometimes a written summary of that patient's condition to the incoming nurse who will assume care for the patient. This summary is called a report and is an important source of data to provide an overview of a patient. Your first task is to get the clinical report on Stephanie Brown. To do this, click **Get Report** in the far right column in this patient's row. From a brief review of this summary, identify the problems and areas of concern that you will need to address for this patient.

When you have finished noting any areas of concern, click on **Go to Nurses' Station**.

■ CHARTS

You can access Stephanie Brown's chart from the Nurses' Station or from the patient's room (304). From the Nurses' Station, click on the chart rack or on the **Chart** icon in the tool bar at the top of your screen. Next, click on the chart labeled **304** to open the medical record for Stephanie Brown. Click on the **Emergency Department** tab to view a record of why this patient was admitted.

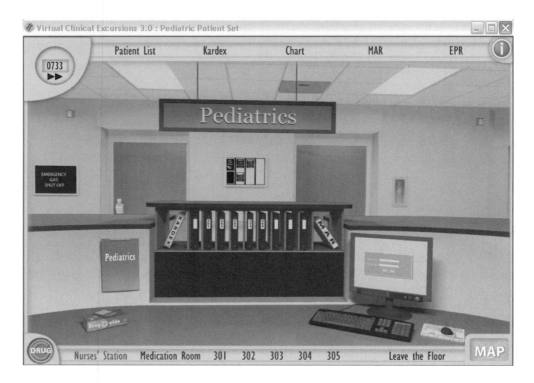

How many days has Stephanie Brown been in the hospital?

What tests were done upon her arrival in the Emergency Department and why?

What was her reason for admission?

You should also click on **Surgical Reports** to learn what procedures were performed and when. Finally, review the **Nursing Admission** and **History and Physical** to learn about the health history of this patient. When you are done reviewing the chart, click **Return to Nurses' Station**.

■ MEDICATIONS

Open the Medication Administration Record (MAR) by clicking on the **MAR** icon in the tool bar at the top of your screen. *Remember:* The MAR automatically opens to the first occupied room number on the floor—which is not necessarily your patient's room number! Since you need to access Stephanie Brown's MAR, click on tab **304** (her room number). Always make sure you are giving the *Right Drug to the Right Patient!*

Examine the list of medications ordered for Stephanie Brown. In the table below, list the medications that need to be given during this period of care (0730-0815). For each medication, note the dosage, route, and time to be given.

Time	Medication	Dosage	Route

Click on **Return to Nurses' Station**. Next, click on **304** on the bottom tool bar and then verify that you are indeed in Stephanie Brown's room. Select **Clinical Alerts** (the icon to the right of Initial Observations) to check for any emerging data that might affect your medication administration priorities. Next, go to the patient's chart (click on the **Chart** icon; then click on **304**). When the chart opens, select the **Physician's Orders** tab.

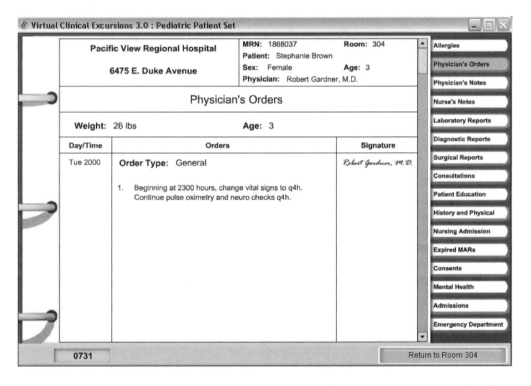

Review the orders. Have any new medications been ordered? Return to the MAR (click **Return to Room 304**; then click **MAR**). Verify that the new medications have been correctly transcribed to the MAR. Mistakes are sometimes made in the transcription process in the hospital setting, and it is sound practice to double-check any new order.

Are there any patient assessments you will need to perform before administering these medications? If so, return to Room 304 and click on **Patient Care** and then **Physical Assessment** to complete those assessments before proceeding.

Now click on the **Medication Room** icon in the tool bar at the bottom of your screen to locate and prepare the medications for Stephanie Brown.

In the Medication Room, you must access the medications for Stephanie Brown from the specific dispensing system in which each medication is stored. Locate each medication that needs to be given in this time period and click on **Put Medication on Tray** as appropriate. (*Hint:* Look in **Unit Dosage** drawer first.) When you are finished, click on **Close Drawer** and then on **View Medication Room**. Now click on the medication tray on the counter on the left side of the medication room screen to begin preparing the medications you have selected. (*Remember:* You can also click **Preparation** in the tool bar at top of the screen.)

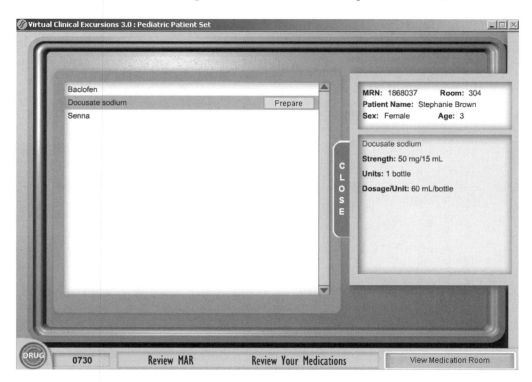

In the preparation area, you should see a list of the medications you put on the tray in the previous steps. Click on the first medication and then click **Prepare**. Follow the onscreen instructions of the Preparation Wizard, providing any data requested. As an example, let's follow the preparation process for docusate sodium, one of the medications due to be administered to Stephanie Brown during this period of care. To begin, click to select **Docusate sodium**; then click **Prepare**. Now work through the Preparation Wizard sequence as detailed below:

Amount of medication in the bottle: 60 mL.
Enter the amount of medication you will draw up into a syringe: **5** mL.
Click **Next**.
Select the patient you wish to set aside the medication for: **Room 304, Stephanie Brown**.
Click **Finish**.
Click **Return to Medication Room**.

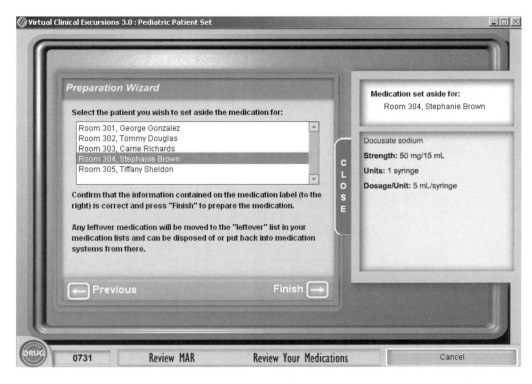

Follow this same basic process for the other medications due to be administered to Stephanie Brown during this period of care. (*Hint:* Look in **IV Storage** and **Automated System**.)

PREPARATION WIZARD EXCEPTIONS

- Some medications in *Virtual Clinical Excursions—Pediatrics* are preprepared by the pharmacy (e.g., IV antibiotics) and taken to the patient room as a whole. This is common practice in most hospitals.
- Blood products are not administered by students through the *Virtual Clinical Excursions—Pediatrics* simulations since blood administration follows specific protocols not covered in this program.
- The *Virtual Clinical Excursions—Pediatrics* simulations do not allow for mixing more than one type of medication, such as regular and Lente insulins, in the same syringe. In the clinical setting, when multiple types of insulin are ordered for a patient, the regular insulin is drawn up first, followed by the longer-acting insulin. Insulin is always administered in a special unit-marked syringe.

Now return to Room 304 (click on **304** on the bottom tool bar) to administer Stephanie Brown's medications.

At any time during the medication administration process, you can perform a further review of systems, take vital signs, check information contained within the chart, or verify patient identity and allergies. Inside Stephanie Brown's room, click **Take Vital Signs**. (*Note:* These findings change over time to reflect the temporal changes you would find in a patient similar to Stephanie Brown.)

When you have gathered all the data you need, click on **Patient Care** and then select **Medication Administration**. Any medications you prepared in the previous steps should be listed on the left side of your screen. Let's continue the administration process with the vancomycin ordered for Stephanie Brown. Click to highlight **Vancomycin** in the list of medications. Next, click on the down arrow to the right of **Select** and choose **Administer** from the drop-down menu. This will activate the Administration Wizard. Complete the Wizard sequence as follows:

- Route: **IV**
- Method: **Intermittent Infusion**
- Site: **Peripheral IV**
- Click **Administer to Patient** arrow.
- Would you like to document this administration in the MAR? **Yes**
- Click **Finish** arrow.

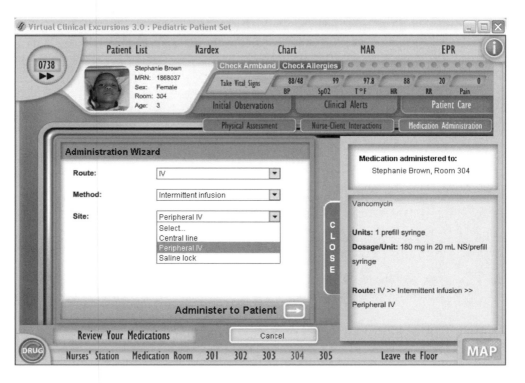

Your selections are recorded by a tracking system and evaluated on a Medication Scorecard stored under Preceptor's Evaluations. This scorecard can be viewed, printed, and given to your instructor. To access the Preceptor's Evaluations, click on **Leave the Floor**. When the Floor Menu appears, select **Look at Your Preceptor's Evaluation**. Then click on **Medication Scorecard** inside the box with Stephanie Brown's name (see example on the following page).

■ MEDICATION SCORECARD

- First, review Table A. Was vancomycin given correctly? Did you give the other medications as ordered?
- Table B shows you which (if any) medications you gave incorrectly.
- Table C addresses the resources used for Stephanie Brown. Did you access the patient's chart, MAR, EPR, or Kardex as needed to make safe medication administration decisions?
- Did you check the patient's armband to verify her identity? Did you check whether your patient had any known allergies to medications? Were vital signs taken?

When you have finished reviewing the scorecard, click **Return to Evaluations** and then **Return to Menu**.

■ VITAL SIGNS

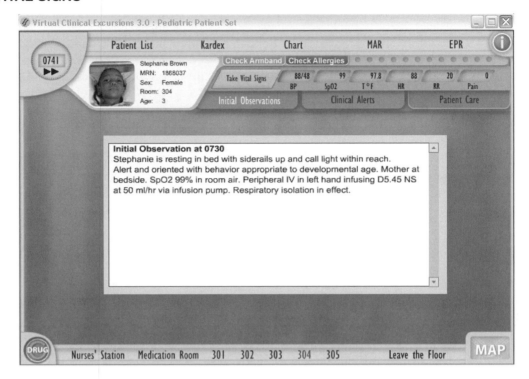

Vital signs, often considered the traditional "signs of life," include body temperature, heart rate, respiratory rate, blood pressure, oxygen saturation of the blood, and pain level.

Inside Stephanie Brown's room, click **Take Vital Signs**. (*Note:* If you are following this detailed tour step by step, you will need to **Restart the Program** from the Floor Menu, sign in again, and navigate to Room 304.) Collect vital signs for this patient and record them below. Note the time at which you collected each of these data. (*Remember:* You can take vital signs at any time. The data change over time to reflect the temporal changes you would find in a patient similar to Stephanie Brown.)

Vital Signs	Findings/Time
Blood pressure	
O₂ saturation	
Heart rate	
Respiratory rate	
Temperature	
Pain rating	

After you are done, click on the **EPR** icon located in the tool bar at the top of the screen. Your username and password are automatically provided. Click on **Login** to enter the EPR. To access Stephanie's records, click on the down arrow next to Patient and choose her room number, **304**. Select **Vital Signs** as the category. Next, in the empty time column on the far right, record the vital signs data you just collected in Stephanie's room. (*Note:* If you need help with this process, see page 16.) Now compare these findings with the data you collected earlier for this patient's vital signs. Use these earlier findings to establish a baseline for each of the vital signs.

    a.   Are any of the data you collected significantly different from the baseline for a particular vital sign?

           Circle One: Yes   No

    b.   If "Yes," which data are different?

■ PHYSICAL ASSESSMENT

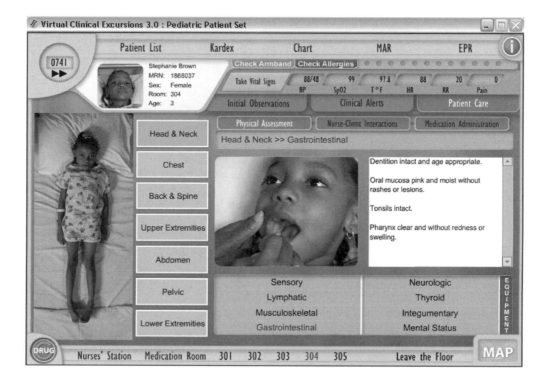

After you have finished examining the EPR for vital signs, click **Exit EPR** to return to Room 304. Click **Patient Care** and then **Physical Assessment**. Think about the information you received in the report at the beginning of this shift, as well as what you may have learned about this patient from the chart. Based on this, what area(s) of examination should you pay most attention to at this time? Is there any equipment you should be monitoring? Conduct a physical assessment of the body areas and systems that you consider priorities for Stephanie Brown. For example, select **Head & Neck**; then click on and assess **Sensory** and **Lymphatic**. Complete any other assessment(s) you think are necessary at this time. In the following table, record the data you collected during this examination.

Area of Examination	Findings
Head & Neck Sensory	
Head & Neck Lymphatic	

After you have finished collecting these data, return to the EPR. Compare the data that were already in the record with those you just collected.

    a. Are any of the data you collected significantly different from the baselines for this patient?

        Circle One: Yes   No

    b. If "Yes," which data are different?

■ **NURSE-CLIENT INTERACTIONS**

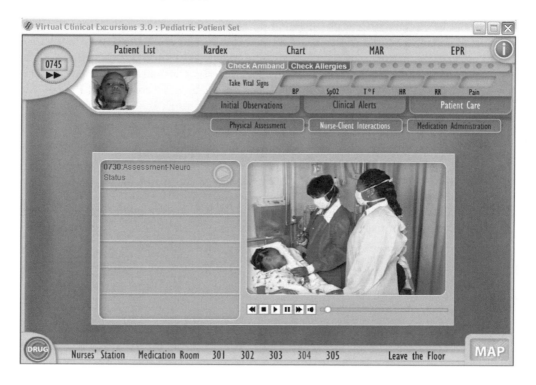

Click on **Patient Care** from inside Stephanie Brown's room (304). Now click on **Nurse-Client Interactions** to access a short video titled **Assessment—Neuro Status**, which is available for viewing at or after 0730 (based on the virtual clock in the upper left corner of your screen; see *Note* below). To begin the video, click on the white arrow next to its title. You will observe a nurse explaining her actions to Stephanie's mother. There are many variations of nursing practice, some exemplifying "best" practice and some not. Note whether the nurse in this interaction displays professional behavior and compassionate care. Are her words congruent with what is going on with the patient? Does this interaction "feel right" to you? If not, how would you handle this situation differently? Explain.

Note: If the video you wish to view is not listed, this means you have not yet reached the correct virtual time to view that video. Check the virtual clock; you may return to access the video once its designated time has occurred—as long as you do so within the same period of care. Or you can click on the fast-forward icon within the virtual clock to advance the time by 2-minute intervals. You will then need to click again on **Patient Care** and **Nurse-Client Interactions** to refresh the screen.

At least one Nurse-Client Interactions video is available during each period of care. Viewing these videos can help you learn more about what is occurring with a patient at a certain time and also prompt you to discern between nurse communications that are ideal and those that need improvement. Compassionate care and the ability to communicate clearly are essential components of delivering quality nursing care, and it is during your clinical time that you will begin to refine these skills.

■ COLLECTING AND EVALUATING DATA

Each of the activities you perform in the Patient Care environment generates a significant amount of assessment data. Remember that after you collect data, you can record your findings in the EPR. You can also review the EPR, patient's chart, videos, and MAR at any time. You will get plenty of practice collecting and then evaluating data in context of the patient's course.

Now, here's an important question for you:

> Did the previous sequence of exercises provide the most efficient way to assess Stephanie Brown?

For example, you went to the patient's room to get vital signs, then back to the EPR to enter data and compare your findings with extant data. Next, you went back to the patient's room to do a physical examination, then again back to the EPR to enter and review data. If this back-and-forth process of data collection and recording seemed inefficient, remember the following:

- Plan all of your nursing activities to maximize efficiency, while at the same time optimizing the quality of patient care. (Think about what data you might need before performing certain tasks. For example, do you need to check a heart rate before administering a cardiac medication or check an IV site before starting an infusion?)

- You collect a tremendous amount of data when you work with a patient. Very few people can accurately remember all these data for more than a few minutes. Develop efficient assessment skills, and record data as soon as possible after collecting them.

- Assessment data are only the starting point for the nursing process.

Make a clear distinction between these first exercises and how you actually provide nursing care. These initial exercises were designed to involve you actively in the use of different software components. This workbook focuses on sensible practices for implementing the nursing process in ways that ensure the highest-quality care of patients.

Most important, remember that a human being changes through time, and that these changes include both the physical and psychosocial facets of a person as a living organism. Think about this for a moment. Some patients may change physically in a very short time (a patient with emerging myocardial infarction) or more slowly (a patient with a chronic illness). Patients' overall physical and psychosocial conditions may improve or deteriorate. They may have effective coping skills and familial support, or they may feel alone and full of despair. In fact, each individual is a complex mix of physical and psychosocial elements, and at least some of these elements usually change through time.

Thus it is crucial that you *DO NOT* think of the nursing process as a simple one-time, five-step procedure consisting of assessment, nursing diagnosis, planning, implementation, and evaluation. Rather, the nursing process should be utilized as a creative and systematic approach to delivering nursing care. Furthermore, because all living organisms are constantly changing, we must apply the nursing process over and over. Each time we follow the nursing process for an individual patient, we refine our understanding of that patient's physical and psychosocial conditions based on collection and analysis of many different types of data. *Virtual Clinical Excursions—Pediatrics* will help you develop both the creativity and the systematic approach needed to become a nurse who is equipped to deliver the highest-quality care to all patients.

REDUCING MEDICATION ERRORS

Earlier in this detailed tour, you learned the basic steps of medication preparation and administration. The following simulations will allow you to practice those skills further—with an increased emphasis on reducing medication errors by using the Medication Scorecard to evaluate your work.

Sign in to work at Pacific View Regional Hospital for Period of Care 2. (*Note:* If you are already working with another patient or during another period of care, click on **Leave the Floor** and then **Restart the Program**; then sign in.)

From the Patient List, select Stephanie Brown. Then click on **Go to Nurses' Station**. Complete the following steps to prepare and administer medications to Stephanie Brown.

- Click on **Medication Room**.
- Click on **MAR** and then on tab **304** to determine prn medications that have been ordered for Stephanie Brown. (*Note:* You may click on **Review MAR** at any time to verify the correct medication order. Always remember to check the patient name on the MAR to make sure you have the correct patient's record—you must click on the correct room number tab within the MAR.) Click on **Return to Medication Room** after reviewing the correct MAR.
- Click on **Unit Dosage** (or on the Unit Dosage cabinet); from the close-up view, click on drawer **304**.
- Select the medications you would like to administer. After each selection, click **Put Medication on Tray**. When you are finished selecting medications, click **Close Drawer** and then **View Medication Room**.
- Click on **Automated System** (or on the Automated System unit itself). Click **Login**.
- On the next screen, specify the correct patient and drawer location.
- Select the medication you would like to administer and click on **Put Medication on Tray**. Repeat this process if you wish to administer other medications from the Automated System.
- When you are finished, click **Close Drawer** and **View Medication Room**.
- From the Medication Room, click on **Preparation** (or on the preparation tray).
- From the list of medications on your tray, highlight the correct medication to administer and click **Prepare**.
- This activates the Preparation Wizard. Supply any requested information; then click **Next**.
- Now select the correct patient to receive this medication and click **Finish**.
- Repeat the previous three steps until all medications that you want to administer are prepared.
- You can click on **Review Your Medications** and then on **Return to Medication Room** when ready. Once you are back in the Medication Room, go directly to Stephanie Brown's room by clicking on **304** at bottom of screen.
- Inside the patient's room, administer the medication, utilizing the six rights of medication administration. After you have collected the appropriate assessment data and are ready for administration, click **Patient Care** and then **Medication Administration**. Verify that the correct patient and medication(s) appear in the left-hand window. Highlight the first medication you wish to administer; then click the down arrow next to Select. From the drop-down menu, select **Administer** and complete the Administration Wizard by providing any information requested. When the Wizard stops asking for information, click **Administer to Patient**. Specify **Yes** when asked whether this administration should be recorded in the MAR. Finally, click **Finish**.

■ SELF-EVALUATION

Now let's see how you did during your medication administration!

- Click on **Leave the Floor** at the bottom of your screen. From the Floor Menu, select **Look at Your Preceptor's Evaluation**. Then click on **Medication Scorecard**.

The following exercises will help you identify medication errors, investigate possible reasons for these errors, and reduce or prevent medication errors in the future.

1. Start by examining Table A. These are the medications you should have given to Stephanie Brown during this period of care. If each of the medications in Table A has a ✓ by it, then you made no errors. Congratulations!

If any medication has an X by it, then you made one or more medication errors.

Compare Tables A and B to determine which of the following types of errors you made: Wrong Dose, Wrong Route/Method/Site, or Wrong Time. Follow these steps:
   a. Find medications in Table A that were given incorrectly.
   b. Now see if those same medications are in Table B, which shows what you actually administered to Stephanie Brown.
   c. Comparing Tables A and B, match the Strength, Dose, Route/Method/Site, and Time for each medication you administered incorrectly.
   d. Then, using the form below, list the medications given incorrectly and mark the errors you made for each medication.

Medication	Strength	Dosage	Route	Method	Site	Time
	❏	❏	❏	❏	❏	❏
	❏	❏	❏	❏	❏	❏
	❏	❏	❏	❏	❏	❏
	❏	❏	❏	❏	❏	❏

2. To help you reduce future medication errors, consider the following list of possible reasons for errors.

- Did not check drug against MAR for correct patient, correct date, correct time, correct drug, and correct dose.
- Did not check drug dose against MAR three times.
- Did not open the unit dose package in the patient's room.
- Did not correctly identify the patient using two identifiers.
- Did not administer the drug on time.
- Did not verify patient allergies.
- Did not check the patient's current condition or vital sign parameters.
- Did not consider why the patient would be receiving this drug.
- Did not question why the drug was in the patient's drawer.
- Did not check the physician's order and/or check with the pharmacist when there was a question about the drug or dose.
- Did not verify that no adverse effects had occurred from a previous dose.

Based on the list of possibilities you just reviewed, determine how you made each error and record the reason in the form below:

Medication	Reason for Error

3. Look again at Table B. Are there medications listed that are not in Table A? If so, you gave a medication to Stephanie Brown that she should not have received. Complete the following exercises to help you understand how such an error might have been made.

   a. Perhaps you gave a medication that was on Stephanie Brown's MAR for this period of care, without recognizing that a change had occurred in the patient's condition, which should have caused you to reconsider. Review patient records as necessary and complete the following form:

Medication	Possible Reasons Not to Give This Medication

   b. Another possibility is that you gave Stephanie Brown a medication that should have been given at a different time. Check her MAR and complete the form below to determine whether you made a Wrong Time error:

Medication	Given to Stephanie Brown at What Time	Should Have Been Given at What Time

c. Maybe you gave another patient's medication to Stephanie Brown. In this case, you made a Wrong Patient error. Check the MARs of other patients and use the form below to determine whether you made this type of error:

Medication	Given to Stephanie Brown	Should Have Been Given to

4. The Medication Scorecard provides some other interesting sources of information. For example, if there is a medication selected for Stephanie Brown but it was not given to her, there will be an X by that medication in Table A, but it will not appear in Table B. In that case, you might have given this medication to some other patient, which is another type of Wrong Patient error. To investigate further, look at Table D, which lists the medications you gave to other patients. See whether you can find any medications ordered for Stephanie Brown that were given to another patient by mistake. However, before you make any decisions, be sure to cross-check the MAR for other patients because the same medication may have been ordered for multiple patients. Use the following form to record your findings:

Medication	Should Have Been Given to Stephanie Brown	Given by Mistake to

5. Now take some time to review the medication exercises you just completed. Use the form below to create an overall analysis of what you have learned. Once again, record each of the medication errors you made, including the type of each error. Then, for each error you made, indicate specifically what you would do differently to prevent this type of error from occurring again.

Medication	Type of Error	Error Prevention Tactic

Submit this form to your instructor if required as a graded assignment, or simply use these exercises to improve your understanding of medication errors and how to reduce them.

Name: _____   Date: _____

The following icons are used throughout this workbook to help you quickly identify particular activities and assignments:

 Indicates a reading assignment—tells you which textbook chapter(s) you should read before starting each lesson

 Indicates a writing activity

 Marks the beginning of an interactive CD-ROM activity—signals you to open or return to your *Virtual Clinical Excursions—Pediatrics* CD-ROM

 Indicates additional CD-ROM instructions

 Indicates questions and activities that require you to consult your textbook

 Indicates the approximate time required to complete an exercise

LESSON 1 ─────────────

Understanding Head Injury

───────────────────────────────

Reading Assignment: Family-Centered Care of the Child During Illness and
Hospitalization (Chapter 21): Intensive Care Unit
The Child with Cerebral Dysfunction (Chapter 28):
Nursing Care of The Unconscious Child; Cerebral Trauma—
Head Injury

Patient: Tommy Douglas, Room 302

Objectives:

1. Evaluate the pathophysiology related to acute head trauma in children.
2. Participate in the care of a comatose child.
3. Review medications given to a child who has experienced a head injury.

Exercise 1

 Writing Activity

 20 minutes

1. What are the clinical symptoms of increased intracranial pressure (ICP) in a child Tommy's
   age and in his condition?

2. List three causes of ICP.

3. Why is the concern for CPP important when caring for a head injury patient?

4. Which of the following vital sign changes are associated with brainstem injury following acute head trauma? Select all that apply.

    _____ Rapid or intermittent respirations

    _____ Wide fluctuations in pulse

    _____ Widening pulse pressure

    _____ Extreme fluctuations in blood pressure

    _____ Elevated temperature

5. One of Tommy's nursing diagnoses is Risk for injury related to physical immobility, depressed sensorium, and intracranial pathology. List four nursing interventions for this nursing diagnosis specific to maintaining a stable ICP.

6. What is the expected outcome related to the nursing diagnosis presented in question 5?

Exercise 2

CD-ROM Activity

 25 minutes

- Sign in to work at Pacific View Regional Hospital for Period of Care 1. (*Note:* If you are already in the virtual hospital from a previous exercise, click on **Leave the Floor** and then **Restart the Program** to get to the sign-in window.)
- From the Patient List, select Tommy Douglas (Room 302).
- Click on **Go to Nurses' Station**.
- Click on **Chart** and then on **302**.
- Select the **Emergency Department** tab and review the ED admission notes.
- While in the chart, also click on and review the **Nurse's Notes** and the **History and Physical.**

   1. What caused Tommy's head injury?

- Now click on **Expired MARs** and review Tommy's expired MAR for Sunday at 2300.
- Next, click on **Physician's Orders** and review orders written in the ED.
- For additional help with the following questions, consult the Drug Guide by first clicking on **Return to Nurses' Station** and then clicking either on the **Drug** icon in the lower left corner of the screen or on the Drug Guide itself on the counter.

   2. Based on your knowledge of head injury, why did Tommy receive mannitol?

   3. Describe the sequence of events from Tommy's admission to the ED to his admission to your unit. (*Hint:* For help, check the Nurse's Notes, Physician's Notes, and Physician's Orders sections of the chart.)

4. List three interventions specific to the treatment of a child with a head injury that were performed before Tommy's arrival on your unit.

Assessing the Head-Injured Patient

 Reading Assignment: Communication and Physical Assessment of the Child
(Chapter 6): Neurologic Assessment
The Child with Cerebral Dysfunction (Chapter 28): Assessment
of Cerebral Function

Patient: Tommy Douglas, Room 302

Objectives:

1. Perform a neurologic assessment on a child who has experienced a head injury.
2. Participate in the care of a comatose child.

Exercise 1

 CD-ROM Activity

35 minutes

- Sign in to work at Pacific View Regional Hospital for Period of Care 1. (*Note:* If you are already in the virtual hospital from a previous exercise, click on **Leave the Floor** and then **Restart the Program** to get to the sign-in window.)
- From the Patient List, select Tommy Douglas (Room 302).
- Click on **Go to Nurses' Station**.
- Click on **Chart** and then on **302** to access Tommy's chart.
- Click on **Emergency Department** and review the admission notes.
- Click on and review the **Nurse's Notes** and the **Physician's Notes**.

1. What are the major components of the Glasgow Coma Scale?

2. In the following table, briefly describe how each of these diagnostic tests is performed. Then provide a rationale for each test to explain its use in assessing the extent of Tommy's head injury. (*Hint:* See Table 28-1 in your textbook and the diagnostic tests found in Tommy's medical record.)

Diagnostic Test	How Test Is Performed	Rationale for Test
Brain CT without contrast		
Skull x-ray		
Cervical spine x-ray (radiograph)		
Brain perfusion test (SPECT)		

Now let's assess Tommy's neurologic status over time since his admission to the ED. To do this, find neurologic assessment data in the following CD-ROM resources; then record your findings in the table as instructed in questions 3 and 4.

- In the patient's chart, click on **Emergency Department** and review this report for Sunday admission.
- Next, click on **Physician's Notes** and review the notes for Monday 0930 and Tuesday 1730.
- Click on **Return to Nurses' Station**.
- Select **EPR** and click on **Login**.
- Specify **302** as the Patient and **Neurologic** as the Category.
- Review the neurologic findings for 0715 Wednesday.

3. In the table below, record the findings from your chart review of Tommy's neurologic status on Sunday, Monday, Tuesday, and Wednesday.

Neurologic Exam	Sunday Admission	Monday 0930	Tuesday 1730	Wednesday 0715
GCS: Total score				
Pupils right: size				
Pupils right: reaction				
Pupils left: size				
Pupils left: reaction				
Cranial nerves I-XII				
Orientation				
Perception and cognition				
Mental status				
Sensory				

- Click on **Exit EPR** and then **Leave the Floor**.
- At the Floor Menu, select **Restart the Program**.
- Sign in for Period of Care 2.
- Again, select Tommy Douglas as your patient and click on **Go to Nurses' Station**.
- Now click on **EPR** and then on **Login**.
- Choose **302** as the Patient and **Neurologic** as the Category. Review the results of the neurologic assessment recorded on Wednesday at 0800.

4. Complete the Glasgow Coma Scale readings below, using the findings from Tommy's neurologic examination at 0800 Wednesday morning.

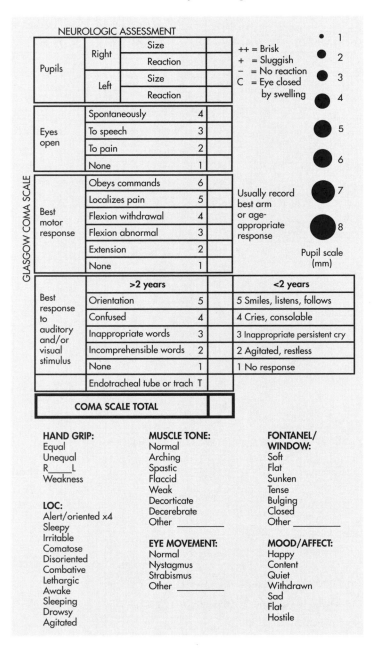

5. How did Tommy's neurologic assessment results change from early in his admission to the PICU (Monday) to his admission to the telemetry unit (Wednesday)? Document your findings below. (*Hint:* Go to the chart and review the Nurse's Notes and Physician's Notes.)

Monday

Wednesday

6. Number the following activities in order of priority, beginning with what you would assess first when examining a critically ill patient such as Tommy.

Activities	Sequence
_____ Check intravenous fluids and lines.	a. 1
_____ Perform a physical assessment.	b. 2
_____ Check ventilator settings.	c. 3
_____ Obtain vital signs.	d. 4

Head Injury Management

Reading Assignment: The Child with Endocrine Dysfunction (Chapter 29): Diabetes Insipidus

Patient: Tommy Douglas, Room 302

Objectives:

1. Analyze laboratory findings associated with acute head injury.
2. Participate in the care of a comatose child.
3. Review medications given to a child who has experienced a head injury.

Exercise 1

 CD-ROM Activity

25 minutes

- Sign in to work at Pacific View Regional Hospital for Period of Care 1. (*Note:* If you are already in the virtual hospital from a previous exercise, click on **Leave the Floor** and then **Restart the Program** to get to the sign-in window.)
- From the Patient List, select Tommy Douglas (Room 302).
- Click on **Go to Nurses' Station**.

1. Which of the following symptoms are commonly associated with diabetes insipidus (DI)? Select all that apply.

_____ Excessive urination

_____ Compensatory insatiable thirst

_____ Dehydration

_____ Electrolyte imbalance

_____ Circulatory collapse

To complete questions 2 through 6, use the following resources on your CD-ROM as needed. (*Remember:* To access the various resources, click on the icons on the toolbar at the top of your screen. When you have finished reviewing one resource and wish to move to another, always look for a navigational button in the lower right corner of your screen—for example, Return to Nurses' Station or Exit EPR.)

- Click on **Chart** and then on **302**. Review the **Nurse's Notes** and **Laboratory Reports**.
- Click on **EPR** and then on **Login**. Choose **302** from the Patient drop-down menu and select various categories as needed.
- Click on **MAR** and then on tab **302** for Tommy's records.

2. List three symptoms of diabetes insipidus that are manifested in Tommy. (*Note:* List specific symptoms such as "Tachycardia: HR greater than 120 bpm.")

3. What medication is being given to Tommy for the treatment of diabetes insipidus?

4. Describe this medication by completing the following table. (*Hint:* Use the Drug Guide as needed.)

Drug	Action	Availability	Dose and Frequency for Children

5. What medications are used as part of Tommy's treatment to assist with blood pressure management? (*Hint:* Check the MAR and the Physician's Orders.)

6. Complete the following table to describe the medications you listed in question 5.
   (*Hint:* Use the Drug Guide as needed.)

Drug	Action	Availability	Dose and Frequency for Children

LESSON 4

Acute Care Phase, Period of Care 1

ᴏᴏ **Reading Assignment:** Family-Centered Care of the Child During Illness and
Hospitalization (Chapter 21): Intensive Care Unit
The Child with Cerebral Dysfunction (Chapter 28): Intracranial
Pressure Monitoring

Patient: Tommy Douglas, Room 302

Objectives:

1. Participate in the care of a comatose child.
2. Perform a neurologic assessment on a child who has experienced a head injury.
3. Review medications given to a child who has experienced a head injury.
4. Interpret assessment findings related to a child whose condition is unstable.

Exercise 1

 CD-ROM Activity

 35 minutes

- Sign in to work at Pacific View Regional Hospital for Period of Care 1. (*Note:* If you are
  already in the virtual hospital from a previous exercise, click on **Leave the Floor** and then
  Restart the Program to get to the sign-in window.)
- From the Patient List, select Tommy Douglas (Room 302).
- Click on **Go to Nurses' Station**.
- Click on **Chart** at the top of the screen or on the rack of charts in the center of the screen.
- Click on **302** for Tommy's chart.
- Click on the **Physician's Orders** and review the orders written Wednesday morning.

1. List three orders written in Tommy's chart that are specific to the treatment of a child with a
   head injury.

• Click on **Return to Nurses' Station**.

• Click on **EPR** and then on **Login**. Choose **302** as the Patient and **Vital Signs** as the Category.

 2. Evaluate Tommy's vital sign results Wednesday at 0700 (just before this shift). Are they normal for his age or his condition at the time? (*Hint:* See the inside back cover of your textbook for vital sign values.)

Now take a current set of vital signs.

 • Click on **Exit EPR** and then on **302** to go to Tommy's room.

• Inside the room, click on **Take Vital Signs**.

3. Record Tommy's current vital signs below.

4. What changes are reflected in the current vital sign findings that indicate a need for prompt intervention?

5. What should be done immediately to prevent further neurologic and systemic deterioration?

6. What should be given first to prevent systemic deterioration? Describe the initial intervention to correct the problem(s) identified in question 4.

• Click on **Chart** and then on **302**.
 • Click on and review the **Physician's Orders**.

7. Which of the orders written at 0730 Wednesday has the most immediate effect on Tommy's blood pressure when implemented?

8. What additional physician orders were written Wednesday morning at 0730 that are directly related to BP stabilization?

 • Click on **Return to Nurses' Station** and then on **Medication Room** at the bottom of your screen.
 • Click on **MAR** to determine what medications Tommy should receive at 0730. (*Note:* You may click on **Review MAR** at any time to verify the correct medication order. Remember to check the patient's name on the MAR to make sure you are viewing the correct record—you must click on the correct room number within the MAR.) Click on **Return to Medication Room** after reviewing the correct MAR.
 • Click on **Unit Dosage** and then on drawer **302**.
 • Click on the medication(s) you would like to administer. For each medication you select, click on **Put Medication on Tray**. When you are finished, click on **Close Drawer**.
 • Click **View Medication Room**.
 • Click on **Automated System** and then on **Login**.
 • Select the correct patient and drawer according to the medication you want to administer. (*Hint:* The automated system is for controlled substances only.) Then click **Open Drawer**.
 • Select the medication(s) you would like to administer, click **Put Medication on Tray**, and then click **Close Drawer**.
 • Click on **View Medication Room**.
 • Begin the preparation process by clicking on **Preparation** at the top of the screen or clicking on the tray on the counter on the left side of the Medication Room.
 • From the list of medications you put on the tray, select the medication you wish to administer; then click **Prepare**.
 • Supply any information requested by the Preparation Wizard; then click **Next**.
 • Choose the correct patient to administer this medication to and click **Finish**.
 • Repeat the above three steps until all medications that you want to administer are prepared.
 • You can click on **Review Your Medications** and then **Return to Medication Room** when ready.

Before you administer Tommy's medications, you must check his existing intravenous lines and the fluids being administered.

- Click on **EPR** and then on **Login**.
- Select **302** as the Patient and **IV** as the Category.
- Review the data recorded on Wednesday at 0700.
- Now click on **Exit EPR**.
- Click on **Chart** and then **302**.
- Select the **Physician's Orders** tab.
- Find the orders for Wednesday at 0600 and review to learn more about the fluids being infused through Tommy's IV lines.

9. Complete the following table to review the types of lines Tommy has and the fluids infusing through each line at 0700 on Wednesday.

Type of Intravenous Line	Location of Intravenous Line	Type of Fluid Infusing and Rationale for Using This Intravenous Line
Central venous line		
Peripheral line		
Arterial line		

- Click on **Exit EPR**.
- Now go to Tommy's room to administer his medication(s) by clicking on **302** at the bottom of the screen.
- Inside the room, click on **Patient Care** and then on **Medication Administration**.
- Next to the medication(s) you want to give, click on **Select** and choose **Administer** from the drop-down menu.
- Complete the Administration Wizard questions; then click on **Administer to Patient**.
- Specify **Yes** to document this to the MAR.
- Finally, click **Finish**.

10. What vital signs would you assess to evaluate the effectiveness of implementing the intervention you identified in question 6?

- Click on **Patient Care** and then on **Nurse-Client Interactions**.
- Select and view the video titled **0800: Intervention—Stabilizing BP**. (*Note:* Check the virtual clock to see whether enough time has elapsed. You can use the fast-forward feature to advance the time by 2-minute intervals if the video is not yet available. Then click again on **Patient Care** and **Nurse-Client Interactions** to refresh the screen.)

The nurse informed Tommy's parents that she would be giving Tommy fluids to help stabilize his blood pressure. Let's jump forward in virtual time to see how effective this intervention was.

- Click on **Leave the Floor**.
- From the Floor Menu, select **Restart the Program**.
- Sign in for Period of Care 2.
- Choose Tommy Douglas as your patient; then click on **Go to Nurses' Station**.
- From the Nurses' Station, click on **EPR** and then on **Login**.
- Choose **302** from the Patient menu and keep **Vital Signs** as the Category.
- Use the left-pointing blue arrow at the bottom of the screen to move back to the data recorded on Wednesday at 0900.

11. What was Tommy's BP at 0900 after the normal saline bolus was administered? Did his blood pressure improve as a result of this intervention?

Acute Care Phase, Period of Care 2

 Reading Assignment: Chronic Illness, Disability, or End-of-Life Care for the Child
and Family (Chapter 18): Perspectives on Care of Children at
the End of Life

Family-Centered Care of the Child During Illness and
Hospitalization (Chapter 21): Intensive Care Unit

The Child with Cerebral Dysfunction (Chapter 28): Altered
States of Consciousness

Appendix C: Common Laboratory Tests

Patient: Tommy Douglas, Room 302

Objectives:

1. Interpret physical assessment findings related to a child whose condition is unstable.
2. Evaluate lab data of the child with a head injury.
3. Observe interactions between health care providers and parents experiencing the loss of a child.

Exercise 1

 CD-ROM Activity

🕐 20 minutes

- Sign in to work at Pacific View Regional Hospital for Period of Care 2. (*Note:* If you are already in the virtual hospital from a previous exercise, click on **Leave the Floor** and then **Restart the Program** to get to the sign-in window.)
- From the Patient List, select Tommy Douglas (Room 302).
- Click on **Get Report.**
- Click on **Go to Nurses' Station**.
- Click on **302**.
- Inside Tommy's room, click on **Take Vital Signs**.

1. Document Tommy's current vital signs in the table below. Also, document these findings in the EPR. (*Hint:* If you need help with the steps for entering data in the EPR, see pp. 15-16 in the **Getting Started** section of this workbook.)

Vital Sign	Findings
T (F)	
Systolic pressure	
Diastolic pressure	
BP mode of measurement	
HR	
RR	
O_2 sat (%)	

→ • Click on **Exit EPR**. In Tommy's room, review the **Initial Observations**.
   • Next, click on **Patient Care**.
   • Choose the various physical assessment areas and appropriate subcategories as needed to complete the table in question 2.

2. Record your findings from Tommy's physical assessment below and on the next page.

Assessment Area	Findings
General Appearance	
HEENT	
Pulmonary	
Cardiovascular	

Assessment	Findings
Gastrointestinal	
Genitourinary	
Musculoskeletal	
Neurologic	

→ • Now click on **Chart**.
  • Click on **302** to access Tommy's chart.
  • Review the **Physician's Orders** for 1100.
  • Then click on **Laboratory Reports** and review the findings for Wednesday morning.

3. In the table below, record Tommy's CBC findings for Wednesday morning. Put an asterisk next to any abnormal findings.

Hematology Laboratory Test	Findings
Hemoglobin	
Hematocrit	
Platelets	

4. What has the physician ordered for Tommy at 1100?

5. What is the most likely rationale for this order, given Tommy's laboratory values at 1100?

6. What other medications are being infused at this same time?

➤ • Still in the Laboratory Reports section, review Tommy's arterial blood gas values (ABGs) for 1100 on Wednesday.

7. Record Tommy's ABGs in the following table.

Arterial Blood Gas Test	Findings—Wednesday 1100
PaO_2	
$PaCO_2$	
pH	
Bicarbonate	

8. Which type of acid-base imbalance is indicated by Tommy's 1100 ABG results?

    a. Metabolic alkalosis
    b. Respiratory alkalosis
    c. Respiratory acidosis
    d. Metabolic acidosis

→ • Review the **Physician's Orders** written for Tommy Douglas at 0820 on Wednesday.

9. What medication was ordered for Tommy at this time?

10. What is the most likely rationale for administering this medication to Tommy?

→ • Click on **Return to Room 302**.
  • Click on **Patient Care** and then **Nurse-Client Interactions**.
  • Select and view the video titled **1115: Family Care Conference**. (*Note:* Check the virtual clock to see whether enough time has elapsed. You can use the fast-forward feature to advance the time by 2-minute intervals if the video is not yet available. Then click again on **Patient Care** and **Nurse-Client Interactions** to refresh the screen.)
  • After viewing the video, click on **Chart** and then on **302**.
  • Review the **Physician's Notes** and **Consultations**.

11. What specific tests did the physicians review with Tommy's parents?

12. What specific findings on physical examination were listed in the consultation notes that concurred with brain death?

13. What is the cold caloric test? (*Hint:* See Neurologic Examination in Chapter 28 in your text-book.)

 • Click on **Return to Room 302**.
• Click on **Patient Care** and then on **Nurse-Client Interactions**.
• Select and view the video titled **1130: Family Care Conference**. (*Note:* Check the virtual clock to see whether enough time has elapsed. You can use the fast-forward feature to advance the time by 2-minute intervals if the video is not yet available. Then click again on **Patient Care** and **Nurse-Client Interactions** to refresh the screen.)

14. What was discussed with Tommy's parents in the 1130 conference?

15. Who was present at the 1115 and 1130 family care conferences?

16. Why is a multidisciplinary team approach important for Tommy's family?

As a follow-up, let's check Tommy's 1300 repeat arterial blood gas results.
 • Click **Leave the Floor**; then select **Restart the Program**.
• Sign in to care for Tommy Douglas during Period of Care 3.
• Click on **Go to Nurses' Station** and then on **Chart**.
• Click on **302** and select **Laboratory Reports**.

17. Below, record Tommy's ABG results for Wednesday at 1300.

Arterial Blood Gas Test	Findings—Wednesday 1300
PaO_2	
$PaCO_2$	
pH	
Bicarbonate	

Acute Care Phase, Period of Care 3

 Reading Assignment: Chronic Illness, Disability, or End-of-Life Care for the Child and Family (Chapter 18): Perspectives on Care of Children at the End of Life; Organ or Tissue Donation/Autopsy; Grief and Mourning

Family-Centered Care of the Child During Illness and Hospitalization (Chapter 21): Intensive Care Unit

The Child with Cerebral Dysfunction (Chapter 28): Cerebral Trauma; Head Injury

Patient: Tommy Douglas, Room 302

Objectives:

1. Interpret physical assessment findings related to a child whose condition is unstable.
2. Evaluate lab data of the child with a head injury.
3. Observe interactions between health care providers and parents experiencing the loss of a child.
4. Describe the diagnostic evaluation necessary to confirm brain death in a child.

Exercise 1

CD-ROM Activity

30 minutes

- Sign in to work at Pacific View Regional Hospital for Period of Care 3. (*Note:* If you are already in the virtual hospital from a previous exercise, click on **Leave the Floor** and then **Restart the Program** to get to the sign-in window.)
- From the Patient List, select Tommy Douglas (Room 302).
- Click on **Go to Nurses' Station**.
- Click on **302** to go to Tommy's room; then click on **Take Vital Signs**.
- Document Tommy's 1500 vital signs results in the EPR. (*Hint:* If you need help entering data in the EPR, see pp. 15-16 in the **Getting Started** section of this workbook.)
- When you have finished entering these data, click on **Exit EPR**.
- Now click on **Chart** and then on **302**.
- Click on **Physician's Orders**.

69

1. Why were new orders written at this time?

 • Review Tommy's chart as needed to answer question 2.

2. In the left column below, list the tests used to establish brain death. In the right column, summarize the results of each of these tests for Tommy.

Diagnostic Test	Findings

 • Click on **Return to Room 302**.
   • Click on **Patient Care** and the **Physical Assessment**.
   • Click on **Head & Neck**.
   • Click on **Neurologic** and complete a neurologic assessment on Tommy.
   • Now click on **EPR** and then on **Login**.
   • Select **302** as the Patient and **Neurologic** as the Category.
   • Review the findings for Wednesday at 1400.

3. Based on your review of the EPR and the in-room neurologic assessment, record Tommy's neurologic findings for Wednesday at 1400 in the table below and on the next page.

Neurologic Assessment	Findings—Wednesday 1400
Glasgow Coma Scale: Eyes	
Glasgow Coma Scale: Verbal	
Glasgow Coma Scale: Motor	
Glasgow Coma Total Score	
Pupils Right: Size	
Pupils Right: Reaction	
Pupils Left: Size	
Pupils Left: Reaction	

Neurologic Assessment	Findings—Wednesday 1400
Cranial Nerves I-XII	
Orientation	
Speech	
Cognitive and Perceptual	
Mental Status	
Sensation	

4. Are your physical examination findings consistent with the physician's and consultants' notes?

5. What is important for the nurse to know when caring for a patient waiting for organ donation? (*Hint:* See Chapter 18 of your textbook.)

→ • Click on **Exit EPR**.

• Once again, observe Tommy's vital signs on Wednesday 1400 by clicking on **Take Vital Signs**.

6. Record Tommy's current vital signs below.

Vital Sign	Findings
T (F)	
Systolic pressure	
Diastolic pressure	
BP mode of measurement	
HR	
RR	
O_2 sat (%)	

7. What do you observe to be continuing problem(s) for Tommy while waiting for organ procurement?

 • Click on **Patient Care** and then **Nurse-Client Interactions**.

• Select and view the video titled **1500: Nurse-Family Communication**. (*Note:* Check the virtual clock to see whether enough time has elapsed. You can use the fast-forward feature to advance the time by 2-minute intervals if the video is not yet available. Then click again on **Patient Care** and **Nurse-Client Interactions** to refresh the screen.)

8. What was reinforced by the nurse during this conversation?

9. Why was it important for the nurse in the video interaction to discuss ways for the family to remember Tommy?

 • Click on **Patient Care** and then **Nurse-Client Interactions**.

• Select and view the video titled **1515: The Grieving Family** to observe the specialist/ family interaction. (*Note:* Check the virtual clock to see whether enough time has elapsed. You can use the fast-forward feature to advance the time by 2-minute intervals if the video is not yet available. Then click again on **Patient Care** and **Nurse-Client Interactions** to refresh the screen.)

10. Describe the role of a child life specialist and explain why this individual is an appropriate choice to meet with Tommy's siblings.

Providing Support for Families Experiencing the Loss of a Child

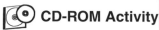 **Reading Assignment:** Chronic Illness, Disability, or End-of-Life Care for the Child and Family (Chapter 18): Perspectives on Care of Children at the End of Life; Organ or Tissue Donation/Autopsy; Grief and Mourning, Decision Making at the End of Life

Patient: Tommy Douglas, Room 302

Objectives:

1. Provide nursing care for the child and family at the end of life.
2. Participate in the multidisciplinary care of the child at the end of life.

Exercise 1

 CD-ROM Activity

45 minutes

- Sign in to work at Pacific View Regional Hospital for Period of Care 2. (*Note:* If you are already in the virtual hospital from a previous exercise, click on **Leave the Floor** and then **Restart the Program** to get to the sign-in window.)
- From the Patient List, select Tommy Douglas (Room 302).
- Click on **Get Report** and read the clinical report.
- Click on **Go to Nurses' Station**.
- Click on **302** to go to Tommy's room.

1. Complete the following table regarding important principles for communicating with families and effective techniques that should be used. (*Hint:* See Table 18-1 and the Guidelines box: Supporting Grieving Families in Chapter 18 in your textbook.)

Communication Approach	Effective Communication Techniques

• Click on **Patient Care** and then on **Nurse-Client Interactions**.

- Select and view the video titled **1115: The Family (Care) Conference**. (*Note:* Check the virtual clock to see whether enough time has elapsed. You can use the fast-forward feature to advance the time by 2-minute intervals if the video is not yet available. Then click again on **Patient Care** and **Nurse-Client Interactions** to refresh the screen.)

2. Complete the table below by identifying what you observed in the family care conference and what you did not observe that you feel you should have.

Communication Approach	Effective Communication Techniques

3. What are the ages of Tommy's siblings?

 4. Based on the ages of Tommy's siblings, describe preschool and school-age children's typical reactions to death and identify possible interventions for support of Tommy's siblings. (*Hint:* See Table 18-3 in your textbook.)

     a. Preschool children

     b. School-age children

• Click on **Chart** and then on **302**.

• Click on **Consultations** and read the Social Services Consult and the Child Life Consult.

5. List at least four interventions found in the consultants' plans that provide an understanding of the health care roles of the following: chaplain, social worker, and child life specialist. Identify the interventions performed by each specific health care professional in this scenario.

 6. Identify at least three strategies discussed in the textbook that can assist nurses and other health care professionals to cope with the loss of a child in their care. (*Hint:* See Chapter 18 in your textbook.)

7. What is nursing burnout? What strategies might you use to prevent this from happening to you?

Tiffany Sheldon

LESSON **8** ———————————————

Anorexia Nervosa: History and Physical Examination

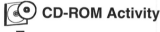 **Reading Assignment:** Health Problems of School-Age Children and Adolescents
(Chapter 17): Anorexia Nervosa

Patient: Tiffany Sheldon, Room 305

Objectives:

1. Identify the early signs of anorexia nervosa.
2. Discuss the special care needs of the adolescent with anorexia nervosa.

Exercise 1

 CD-ROM Activity

🕐 25 minutes

- Sign in to work at Pacific View Regional Hospital for Period of Care 1. (*Note:* If you are already in the virtual hospital from a previous exercise, click on **Leave the Floor** and then **Restart the Program** to get to the sign-in window.)
- From the Patient List, select Tiffany Sheldon (Room 305).
- Click on **Go to Nurses' Station**.
- Click on **Chart** and then on **305**.
- Click on **Emergency Department** and review the report.

1. Describe Tiffany's past illness history leading up to her ED visit.

2. List the three treatment goals for patients with anorexia nervosa (AN) as cited in the text-
    book.

→ • While still in the chart, click on **Nursing Admission**.

   3. Review the Nursing Admission and list three family stressors found in Tiffany's family.

→ • Now click on **Physician's Orders**.
   • Note Tiffany's medical diagnosis documented on the Physician's Orders for 0600 Wednesday.
   • Click on **Return to Nurses' Station**.
   • Click on **305** to enter Tiffany's room.
   • Click on **Patient Care** and then **Physical Assessment**.
   • Perform a focused physical assessment on Tiffany.

   4. List six findings from the physical assessment that relate to Tiffany's diagnosis of malnutri-
      tion.

5. Based on the ED admission data and Tiffany Sheldon's past and present health history, list three appropriate nursing diagnoses with the etiology statement included.

6. What was Tiffany's weight on admission to the ED?

7. What is Tiffany's height? (*Hint:* Review the Nursing Admission in the chart.)

8. Using the CDC growth chart on the next page (Body mass index-for-age percentiles: Girls, 2 to 20 years), plot Tiffany's body mass index of 13.8 kg/m^2 according to her age: (weight in pounds/height in inches) / height in inches × 703. At what percentile is her BMI?

CDC Growth Charts: United States

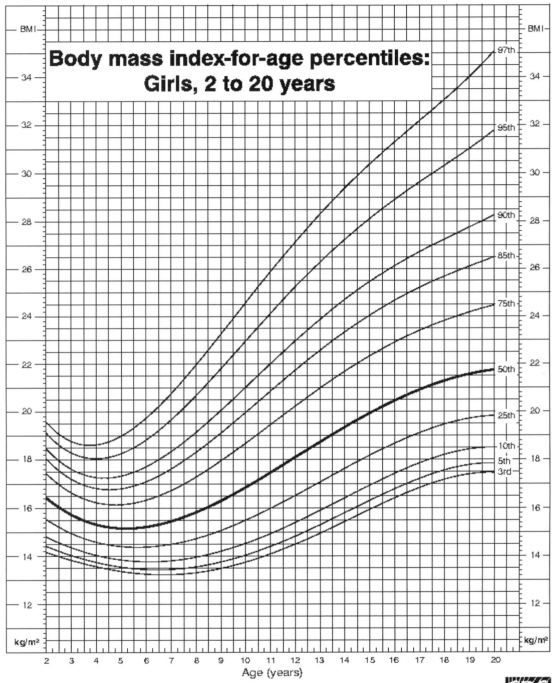

Body mass index-for-age percentiles: Girls, 2 to 20 years

Age (years)

Published May 30, 2000.
SOURCE: Developed by the National Center for Health Statistics in collaboration with
the National Center for Chronic Disease Prevention and Health Promotion (2000).

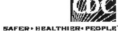

Pathophysiology of Anorexia Nervosa

/O7O **Reading Assignment:** Health Problems of School-Age Children and Adolescents
(Chapter 17): Anorexia Nervosa

Patient: Tiffany Sheldon, Room 305

Objectives:

1. Distinguish between the two types of anorexia nervosa (AN).
2. Describe physical and behavioral characteristics of the adolescent with AN.
3. Describe the DSM-IV diagnostic criteria for AN in relation to Tiffany Sheldon's presentation.

Exercise 1

 CD-ROM Activity

 25 minutes

- Sign in to work at Pacific View Regional Hospital for Period of Care 1. (*Note:* If you are already in the virtual hospital from a previous exercise, click on **Leave the Floor** and then **Restart the Program** to get to the sign-in window.)
- From the Patient List, select Tiffany Sheldon (Room 305).
- Click on **Go to Nurses' Station**.
- Click on **Chart** and then on **305**.
- Click on **History and Physical**.

1. Based on the H&P, which type of anorexia nervosa does Tiffany have? Explain your answer based on Tiffany's recent history as reported by her mother.

2. What is the average age of onset of anorexia nervosa?

   a. 10-25 years with a mean of 13 years
   b. 12-18 years with a mean of 16.8 years
   c. 8-16 years with a mean of 14 years
   d. 12-20 years with a mean of 15.25 years

3. What are some personality characteristics found in children with anorexia nervosa?

   a. Perfectionism, high achievement in academics, conformity, and conscientiousness
   b. Fearful, dependent, and controlling
   c. Goal-oriented, physically active, with erratic behaviors
   d. All of the above

4. All of the following are psychological characteristics of anorexia nervosa *except*:

   a. pursuit of thinness.
   b. fear of fatness.
   c. disordered body perception.
   d. response to traumatic or personal life events.
   e. response to teasing, life changes.
   f. sequelae of infectious diseases.

For questions 5 through 10, circle either True or False. For any statements you identify as false, provide a rationale for your decision.

5. Young people involved in competitive sports or activities such as ballet and gymnastics are also at risk for unsafe weight control practices and eating disorders such as anorexia nervosa.

   True / False

6. Anorexia nervosa is more common in females.

   True / False

7. Females typically have a more difficult clinical course than males who are diagnosed with anorexia nervosa.

     True / False

8. Complete recovery rates for anorexia nervosa are very favorable.

     True / False

9. Physical changes associated with anorexia nervosa are reversible with adequate nutrition and leave no sequelae.

     True / False

10. The prognosis is best for those in whom anorexia nervosa is diagnosed at a relatively early age, before abnormal eating patterns and other weight-loss techniques are established and emaciation has set in.

     True / False

10 ——————————————

Anorexia Nervosa: Clinical Signs and Symptoms

————————————————————————————

Reading Assignment: Communication and Physical Assessment of the Child
(Chapter 6): Evaluation of Nutritional Assessment;
Table 6-1 (Clinical Assessment of Nutritional Status);
Physical Examination—Skin

Patient: Tiffany Sheldon, Room 305

Objectives:

1. Identify the physical assessment characteristics of a child with anorexia nervosa.
2. Recognize potentially life-threatening physical assessment findings in the child with anorexia nervosa.
3. Identify diagnostic laboratory values indicative of dehydration.

Exercise 1

 CD-ROM Activity

 30 minutes

- Sign in to work at Pacific View Regional Hospital for Period of Care 1. (*Note:* If you are already in the virtual hospital from a previous exercise, click on **Leave the Floor** and then **Restart the Program** to get to the sign-in window.)
- From the Patient List, select Tiffany Sheldon (Room 305).
- Click on **Go to Nurses' Station**.
- Click on **Chart** and then on **305**.
- Click on **Emergency Department**.

1. The Review of Systems in the ED revealed the findings in the right column below. Match each finding with the corresponding body system.

System	Finding
_____ Integumentary	a. Upper and lower extremity weakness
_____ Cardiovascular	b. 4-second capillary refill and 1+ pedal edema
_____ Genitourinary	c. Decreased skin turgor and dry skin
_____ Gastrointestinal	d. Constipation
_____ Neuromuscular	e. Decreased urine output

2. List the clinical findings of Tiffany's physical examination documented by the nurse and physician in the ED.

3. Identify initial clinical findings in the ED record that require immediate attention.

 4. Describe the most likely cause of the findings you identified in question 3, as well as the significance of the findings. (*Hint:* See Dehydration in Chapter 24 of your textbook.)

 • Click on **Return to Nurses' Station**.
- Click on **305** to go to Tiffany's room.
- Click on **Patient Care** and then **Nurse-Client Interactions**.
- Select and view the video titled **0730: Initial Assessment**. (*Note:* Check the virtual clock to see whether enough time has elapsed. You can use the fast-forward feature to advance the time by 2-minute intervals if the video is not yet available. Then click again on **Patient Care** and **Nurse-Client Interactions** to refresh the screen.)

5. In the video, what assessment does the nurse perform related to Tiffany's cardiovascular status?

6. What else does the nurse ask Tiffany in the video interaction that represents cardiovascular assessment?

- Click on **Chart** and then **305**.
- Select **Laboratory Reports**.
- Review the findings documented in the ED on Wednesday at 0530.

7. Below, record Tiffany's laboratory results obtained in the ED. For each test, provide the normal range of values for a child Tiffany's age (14). (*Hint:* See Appendix E in your textbook.)

Test	Tiffany's Result	Normal Range
Glucose		
Sodium		
Potassium		
Chloride		
Creatinine—serum		
BUN		
Calcium—serum, total		
Protein—serum		
Albumin—serum		

8. Tiffany's initial specific gravity is 1.035. What does specific gravity measure? What is the significance of this clinical finding in relation to Tiffany's clinical status?

→ • Now click on and review the initial **Physician's Orders**.

9. Tiffany is being treated for dehydration. What laboratory tests are ordered to assess and monitor the status of her dehydration?

    a. Albumin, protein, and alkaline phosphatase
    b. HCG urinalysis and specific gravity
    c. Glucose, phosphorus, calcium, and magnesium
    d. BUN, creatinine, Chem 7, and specific gravity

10. What is the purpose of obtaining a urine HCG on Tiffany? What does the test reveal?

11. Tiffany has been diagnosed with malnutrition. What laboratory tests are ordered to assess and monitor her malnutrition?

    a. Serum VDRL, specific gravity, and alkaline phosphatase
    b. Protein, albumin, glucose, and alkaline phosphatase
    c. Protein, calcium, ALT, and AST
    d. Chem 7, protein, and BUN

12. Tiffany has been diagnosed with bradycardia. What laboratory tests assess and monitor her cardiac function?

    a. BUN, creatinine, protein, and glucose
    b. Chem 7, VDRL, specific gravity, and alkaline phosphatase
    c. Chem 7, phosphorus, calcium, and magnesium
    d. ALT, AST, urine specific gravity, and protein

→ • Next, click on **Nursing Admission** and review.

13. For which of the following risks was Tiffany Sheldon assessed on admission? Select all that apply.

    _____ Risk for infection

    _____ Risk for hypertension

    _____ Risk for falls

    _____ Risk for impaired tissue integrity

14. What is the underlying cause of these assessed risks?

    a. Poor nutrition, electrolyte imbalance, and muscle wasting
    b. Poor nutrition, depression, and too much exercise
    c. Amenorrhea, electrolyte imbalance, and depression
    d. Muscle wasting, depression, and too much exercise

15. What is the best explanation for the finding of lanugo in Tiffany's physical exam?

    a. Hair follicles are starved of the appropriate nutrition needed to produce healthy hair.
    b. It is the result of cold intolerance in an attempt to warm the body.
    c. It is secondary to cardiac insufficiency.
    d. All of the above explain Tiffany's findings.

16. For which of the following reasons should rapid weight gain, also referred to as refeeding syndrome, be avoided in patients with anorexia nervosa? Select all that apply.

    _____   It has been associated with severe metabolic abnormalities.

    _____   Cardiovascular overload has led to death in patients with anorexia nervosa.

    _____   Patients with anorexia nervosa are fearful of gaining weight.

    _____   Patients with anorexia nervosa have a distorted body image.

17. Urinary tract problems are frequent in patients with anorexia nervosa, including the presence of ketones and proteins in the urine. What is the most likely cause of these findings?

    a. Low body temperature
    b. Fat and protein breakdown
    c. Decreased cardiac output

18. To which of the following is Tiffany's complaint of constipation related? Select all that apply.

    _____   Delayed gastric emptying

    _____   Decreased fluid intake

    _____   Muscle wasting

    _____   Reduced intestinal motility

19. Which of the following physical symptoms of anorexia nervosa does Tiffany not have? (Select all that apply.)

    _____   Lowered body temperature

    _____   Bradycardia

    _____   Decreased blood pressure

    _____   Cold intolerance

    _____   Headaches

    _____   Vomiting

    _____   Secondary amenorrhea

20. What best explains the finding of edema on Tiffany's admission?

21. List two lab values from question 7 that are helpful in evaluating the malnourished patient.

11

Management of Anorexia Nervosa

 Reading Assignment: Health Problems of School-Age Children and Adolescents (Chapter 17): Anorexia Nervosa

Patient: Tiffany Sheldon, Room 305

Objectives:

1. Identify the contents and goal of the behavioral contract, or "eating contract."
2. List priority goals in the treatment of anorexia nervosa.
3. Describe the role of the multidisciplinary health care team in the management of anorexia nervosa.

Exercise 1

Writing Activity

5 minutes

1. Which of the following are goals of treatment for anorexia nervosa? Select all that apply.

_____ Reinstitution of normal nutrition or reversal of the severe state of malnutrition

_____ Resolution of disturbed patterns of family interaction

_____ Individual psychotherapy to correct deficits and distortions of psychologic functioning

_____ Neurologic assessment to evaluate for physical therapy

Exercise 2

 CD-ROM Activity

🕐 25 minutes

Note: For this exercise, you will need to observe and consider four video interactions in two different periods of care before answering questions. Therefore you may wish to review questions 1 through 8 before signing in and then take notes while you view the videos.

• Sign in to work at Pacific View Regional Hospital for Period of Care 2. (*Note:* If you are already in the virtual hospital from a previous exercise, click on **Leave the Floor** and then **Restart the Program** to get to the sign-in window.)
• From the Patient List, select Tiffany Sheldon (Room 305).
• Click on **Go to Nurses' Station**.
• Click on **305** to go to Tiffany's room.

For the first video:

• Click on **Patient Care** and then on **Nurse-Client Interactions**.
• Select and view the video titled **1115: Managing Anorexia Nervosa**. (*Note:* Check the virtual clock to see whether enough time has elapsed. You can use the fast-forward feature to advance the time by 2-minute intervals if the video is not yet available. Then click again on **Patient Care** and **Nurse-Client Interactions** to refresh the screen.)

For the second video:

• Click again on **Patient Care** and then **Nurse-Client Interactions**.
• View the video titled **1130: Monitoring Compliance**.
• When you have finished viewing this video, click on **Leave the Floor**.
• At the Floor Menu, select **Restart the Program**.

For the third video:

• Sign in again to care for Tiffany Sheldon, this time for Period of Care 3.
• Click on **Go to Nurses' Station** and then on **305**.
• Again, click on **Patient Care** and then on **Nurse-Client Interactions**.
• Select and view the video titled **1500: Relapse—Contributing Factors**.

For the fourth video:

• Click again on **Patient Care** and then **Nurse-Client Interactions**.
• Select and view the video titled **1530: Facilitating Success**.
• After watching this fourth video interaction, complete questions 1 through 8.

  1. List four items that Tiffany has agreed to in her eating contract.

2. What statement does Tiffany make during the video interactions that may lead you to believe she has concerns about her weight (disordered eating) and caloric intake?

3. Is the targeted caloric intake goal of 2100 kcal for Tiffany within the therapeutic range according to the textbook?

4. What is the expected daily weight gain projected for a patient with anorexia nervosa?

5. What possible rationale might the nurse have for asking Tiffany's mother if she may speak to Tiffany alone?

6. What behavioral modification plans are implemented and discussed with Tiffany? What are these plans specifically designed to monitor?

7. What purpose would monitoring Tiffany in the bathroom serve in regard to food intake?

8. The precise cause of anorexia nervosa is unknown; however, recommendations for management have suggested that treatment is best managed by an interdisciplinary team. Ideally, which of the following should be included on the team? Select all that apply.

_____ Dietitians

_____ Physicians and nurses

_____ Counselors

_____ Psychologists or psychiatrists

For questions 9 through 13, circle either True or False. For any statement you identify as false, provide a rationale for your decision.

9. The self-damaging behaviors of AN are a result of the patient's distorted body image and self-awareness, feelings of self-doubt, ineffectiveness, helplessness, and lack of control.

   True / False

10. Individual team members can make alterations to the plan based on their individual interactions with the patient.

    True / False

11. If the patient views the behavioral plan as coercive and becomes depressed by the approach, it is possible that weight gain may not be sustained outside the hospital.

    True / False

12. Family therapy needs to be directed toward disengagement and redirection of malfunctioning processes in the family.

    True / False

13. Prevention of AN is very straightforward and usually very effective.

    True / False

12

Nursing Care of the Child with Anorexia Nervosa

✍ **Reading Assignment:** Health Problems of School-Age Children and Adolescents
(Chapter 17): Anorexia Nervosa

Patient: Tiffany Sheldon, Room 305

Objectives:

1. Identify the contents and goal of the behavioral contract, or "eating contract."
2. Describe the psychologic implications of food intake in relation to perceived body image in the adolescent with anorexia nervosa.

 Exercise 1

 CD-ROM Activity

20 minutes

- Sign in to work at Pacific View Regional Hospital for Period of Care 2. (*Note:* If you are already in the virtual hospital from a previous exercise, click on **Leave the Floor** and then **Restart the Program** to get to the sign-in window.)
- From the Patient List, select Tiffany Sheldon (Room 305).
- Click on **Go to Nurses' Station**.
- Click on **Chart** and then on **305**.
- Click on **Consultations**.
- Review the Nutrition Consult at 1100.
- Click on **Return to Nurses' Station** and then on **305** to go to Tiffany's room.
- Click on **Patient Care** and then on **Nurse-Client Interactions**.
- Select and view the video titled **1115: Managing Anorexia Nervosa**. (*Note:* Check the virtual clock to see whether enough time has elapsed. You can use the fast-forward feature to advance the time by 2-minute intervals if the video is not yet available. Then click again on **Patient Care** and **Nurse-Client Interactions** to refresh the screen.)
- Next, select and view the video titled **1130: Monitoring Compliance**.

95

1. The dietitian has been working with Tiffany and is aware of her history. In the 1115 video interaction, what is the purpose of the visit with Tiffany? Select all that apply.

    _____   To develop the eating contract

    _____   To get Tiffany's agreement about the eating contract

    _____   To assess Tiffany's current nutritional status

    _____   To present Tiffany with a menu to help in selection of a diet

2. What concern does Tiffany express during the video interaction with the dietitian?

    a. She is concerned about when she will be discharged from the hospital.
    b. She is concerned that she will not be able to consume all the calories in the contract.
    c. She is concerned that the diet will make her more constipated.
    d. She is concerned that the diet will make her gain weight too quickly.

3. What are possible barriers to Tiffany being successful in negotiating the eating contract?

    a. Difficulty thinking clearly because of her poor nutritional status
    b. Inability to find hospital foods that are acceptable to her
    c. Unwillingness to remain in the hospital
    d. Concern about missing school

4. The dietitian is working with a treatment team to help monitor progress. What is the most important medical risk involved in developing a nutritional plan for Tiffany?

    a. Possible physical injury from too much exercise
    b. Worsening constipation from increasing the diet
    c. Complications of refeeding syndrome, leading to severe metabolic abnormalities and cardiac complications

→ • Click on **Chart**.
    • Click on **305** for Tiffany's chart.
    • Click on **Consultations** and review the Psychiatric Consult at 1500 on Wednesday.

5. What are the main goals of psychotherapy in the adolescent with AN? Select all that apply.

    _____   To promote the correction of metabolic abnormalities

    _____   To support the eating contract and help the patient understand the illness

    _____   To develop a therapeutic alliance to permit open discussion of the patient's feelings and help develop more appropriate ways to communicate and cope

    _____   To provide individual cognitive therapy to deal with environmental, familial, and personal conditions that may lead to anorexia nervosa

6. Identify three underlying issues that the psychiatrist identifies as contributing factors in Tiffany's illness.

For questions 7 through 10, circle either True or False. For any statement you identify as false, provide a rationale for your decision.

7. An additional purpose for psychotherapy in anorexia nervosa is to help the patient develop a locus of control in order to express herself in acceptable ways.

   True / False

8. Daily exercise is an important part of the recovery plan and a way to relieve stress.

   True / False

9. It is important for the patient to understand that the team is in control of the contract and that the patient must obey all parts of the contract without question.

   True / False

10. It is important to provide family members with support to help them deal with the pressures of managing a patient with anorexia nervosa.

    True / False

Stephanie Brown

Emergent Nursing Care of the Child with Meningitis

Reading Assignment: Communication and Physical Assessment of the Child (Chapter 6): Neurologic Assessment

The Child with Cerebral Dysfunction (Chapter 28): Cerebral Dysfunction; Increased Intracranial Pressure; Intracranial Pressure Monitoring; Bacterial and Aseptic Meningitis

Patient: Stephanie Brown, Room 304

Objectives:

1. Analyze laboratory findings associated with childhood meningitis.
2. Differentiate between bacterial and aseptic meningitis.
3. Describe the components of a neurologic assessment for a child who is diagnosed with meningitis.
4. Describe the pathophysiology of meningitis.

Exercise 1

Clinical Preparation: Writing Activity

 5 minutes

1. Match the following terms with the corresponding characteristics.

Term	Characteristic
_____ Meningitis	a. Viral inflammation of the meninges
_____ Mode of meningitis transmission	b. Greatest morbidity between birth and 4 years
_____ Bacterial meningitis	c. Vascular dissemination of mucosal organisms frequently from the nasopharyngeal site
_____ Predisposition to meningitis	d. Pyogenic inflammation of the meninges
_____ Aseptic meningitis	e. Inflammation of the membranes covering the brain and spinal cord

2. What are common clinical manifestations of meningitis in children and adolescents?

Exercise 2

 CD-ROM Activity

 45 minutes

- Sign in to work at Pacific View Regional Hospital for Period of Care 1. (*Note:* If you are already in the virtual hospital from a previous exercise, click on **Leave the Floor** and then **Restart the Program** to get to the sign-in window.)
- From the Patient List, select Stephanie Brown (Room 304).
- Click on **Go to Nurses' Station**.
- Click on **304** to go to Stephanie's room.
- Click on **Patient Care** and then **Physical Assessment**.
- Click on **Head & Neck**.
- Click on **Neurologic** and view the assessment.

 1. State the physiologic basis for Stephanie's headache. (*Hint:* See Increased Intracranial Pressure in Chapter 28 in the textbook.)

 • Click on **Chart**.
- Click on **304** to view Stephanie's Chart.
- Click on **Emergency Department** and review.
- Then click on and read the **Nurse's Notes** and **Physician's Notes**.

2. List the clinical manifestations of meningitis exhibited by Stephanie in the ED.

• Click on and read the **History and Physical** section of Stephanie's chart.

    3. Describe the Glasgow Coma Scale and list the three-part assessment of the coma scale.

 • Click on **Laboratory Reports**. Review the findings recorded in the ED on Monday at 0100.

 4. Below, list the abnormal findings you noted for Stephanie Brown in the Laboratory Reports. For each abnormal finding, give the normal range of results. Finally, what does each finding indicate? (*Hint:* Common laboratory tests are in Appendix C of the textbook).

Lab Test	Abnormal Results	Normal Range	Indications

• Now click on **Diagnostic Reports** and review the summary of Stephanie's lumbar puncture.

5. When a child has suspected meningitis, spinal fluid pressure can be measured during the lumbar puncture with a manometer. What is Stephanie's spinal fluid pressure? What is the significance of these results in relation to Stephanie's condition? (*Hint:* The normal range for a child her age is 60-100 mm H_2O.)

 6. Below, list each of the cerebral spinal fluid (CSF) results from Stephanie's lumbar puncture on Monday. For each finding, give the normal range of results and identify what each finding indicates. (*Hint:* Common laboratory tests are in Appendix C of the textbook.)

CSF (Lumbar)	Results	Normal Range	Indications

7. What is the rationale for placing Stephanie in respiratory isolation?

 • Click on **Physician's Orders** and review.

8. What medication is ordered for Stephanie for a high temperature?

9. What is the rationale for administering this medication by rectum (PR) in the ED at 0100 on Monday?

10. What is the rationale for having the head of Stephanie's bed elevated 45 degrees?

11. Describe the standard isolation technique for a child with meningitis in an acute care center. (*Note:* You may describe the standard practice in an institution where you work as staff member or student.)

12. What is the physiologic basis for giving Stephanie a normal saline bolus in the ED? (*Hint:* See the Systems Review section of the Emergency Department Record in the chart.)

→ • Click on **Return to Room 304**.
   • Click on **MAR** and review Stephanie's records.

13. An intravenous infusion is started immediately in a child with suspected meningitis to administer IV fluids and:

   a. antiepileptic drugs.
   b. steroid drugs.
   c. blood products.
   d. antimicrobial drugs.

14. Give a rationale for your answer to question 13.

Now let's go to the Medication Room and prepare to administer all of the 0730 and 0800 medications ordered for Stephanie.

- First, click on **Return to Room 304**.
- Next, click on **Medication Room**.
- Click on **MAR** to determine what medications Stephanie should receive for 0730 and 0800. You may review the MAR at any time to verify the correct medication order. (*Hint:* Remember to look at the patient name on the MAR to make sure you have the correct record—you must click on the tab with Stephanie's room number within the MAR.) Click on **Return to Medication Room** after reviewing the correct MAR.
- Click on **Unit Dosage** and then on drawer **304**.
- Select the medications you would like to administer. For each medication you select, click on **Put Medication on Tray**. When you are finished, click on **Close Drawer**.
- Click **View Medication Room**.
- Now click on **Automated System** and **Login**.
- Select the correct patient and drawer according to the medication you want to administer. (*Hint:* This automated system is for controlled substances only.) Then click **Open Drawer**.
- Select the medication you would like to administer, click on **Put Medication on Tray**, and then click **Close Drawer**.
- Click **View Medication Room**.
- Click on **Preparation** and select the medication to administer.
- Click **Prepare** and wait for the Preparation Wizard to appear. If the Wizard requests information, provide your answer(s) and then click **Next**.
- Choose the correct patient and then click **Finish**.
- Repeat the previous three steps until all medications that you want to administer are prepared.
- You can click on **Review Your Medications** and then click **Return to Medication Room** when ready. Once you are back in the Medication Room, go directly to Stephanie Brown's room by clicking on **304** at the bottom of the screen.
- In Stephanie Brown's room, administer the medications, using the five rights of medication administration. After you have collected the appropriate assessment data and are ready for administration, click **Patient Care** and then **Medication Administration**. Verify that the correct patient and medication(s) appear in the left-hand window. Then click the down arrow next to Select. From the drop-down menu, select **Administer** and complete the Administration Wizard by providing any information requested. When the Wizard stops asking for infor-

mation, click **Administer to Patient**. Specify **Yes** when asked whether this administration should be recorded in the MAR. Finally, click **Finish**. Complete these steps for each medication you wish to administer.

15. In the mock MAR form below, document the medications you administered.

Medication/Dose	2300-0700	0700-1500	1500-2300

16. Stephanie is receiving maintenance IV fluids with strict intake and output to prevent what severe complication?

• To answer questions 17 through 19, you will need to consult the Drug Guide provided on the CD-ROM.

• To access the Drug Guide, click on the **Drug** icon in the lower left corner of your screen. When the Drug Guide opens, use the Search bar or scroll through the alphabetic list of drugs at the top of the screen; select **vancomycin**.

17. Provide the rationale for the intravenous administration of this drug (versus oral administration).

18. Briefly describe the procedure for administering vancomycin intravenously to a child Stephanie's age. Include the correct dilution, if required.

19. List three serious side effects for which the nurse should be vigilant during and after the administration of this medication.

Now let's see how you did administering Stephanie's medications.

 • Click on **Leave the Floor** at the bottom of your screen. From the Floor Menu, select **Look at Your Preceptor's Evaluation**. Then click on **Medication Scorecard.**

• Review the scorecard to see whether or not you correctly administered the appropriate medication(s). If not, why do you think you were incorrect? According to Table C in this scorecard, what resources should have been used and what important assessments should have been completed before administering the medication(s)? Did you use these resources and perform these assessments correctly?

• Print a copy of the Medication Scorecard for your instructor to evaluate.

Nursing Care of the Hospitalized Child

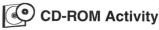 **Reading Assignment:** The Child with Gastrointestinal Dysfunction (Chapter 24): Constipation

The Child with Cerebral Dysfunction (Chapter 28): Bacterial Meningitis

Patient: Stephanie Brown, Room 304

Objectives:

1. Describe the nursing care of the child with meningitis and constipation.
2. Identify the rationale for auditory testing in the child with meningitis.

Exercise 1

CD-ROM Activity

45 minutes

- Sign in to work at Pacific View Regional Hospital for Period of Care 2. (*Note:* If you are already in the virtual hospital from a previous exercise, click on **Leave the Floor** and then **Restart the Program** to get to the sign-in window.)
- From the Patient List, select Stephanie Brown (Room 304).
- Click on **Go to Nurses' Station**.
- Click on **Chart** and then on **304**.
- Click on **Emergency Department** and review this report.
- Click on and review the **Physician's Orders** and **Physician's Notes** for Wednesday at 0900.
- Click on **Return to Nurses' Station**.
- Click on **304** to go to Stephanie's room.
- Click **Patient Care** and then on **Nurse-Client Interactions**.
- Select and view the video titled **1120: Preventing Spread of Disease**. (*Note:* Check the virtual clock to see whether enough time has elapsed. You can use the fast-forward feature to advance the time by 2-minute intervals if the video is not yet available. Then click again on **Patient Care** and **Nurse-Client Interactions** to refresh the screen.)

1. What might explain why the physician decreased Stephanie's IV rate to 10 mL/hr?

2. How did Stephanie's nurse explain the basis for the respiratory isolation?

3. Based on your earlier review of the Physician's Notes, what was the physician's most likely rationale for discontinuing the respiratory isolation and vancomycin for Stephanie?

→ • Still in Stephanie's room, click on **Clinical Alerts** and review.

4. What does the Clinical Alert say regarding Stephanie's abdominal assessment?

5. When did Stephanie have her last bowel movement?

• Return to Stephanie's chart and review the **Physician's Notes** to answer question 6.

 6. Compare the Monday and Wednesday notes in regard to the Kernig sign, Brudzinski sign, and nuchal rigidity results for Stephanie. Record any changes below. (*Hint:* See Clinical Manifestations in Chapter 28 of your textbook.)

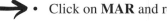 • Click on **MAR** and review Stephanie's medication orders.

7. Are there further indications for performing an audiogram on this patient (besides the diagnosis of meningitis)?

 • Click on **Return to Room 304**.
 • Click on **Chart** and then on **304**.
 • Click on **Physician's Orders** and review the orders for 1100 on Wednesday.

8. What medication is ordered for Stephanie at this time?

 • Click on **Return to Room 304**.
 • Click on the **Drug** icon in the lower left corner of your screen. Locate and review the information for the drug ordered for Stephanie.

9. Complete the following table for the drug you identified in question 8. Relate your answers specifically to Stephanie's need for the medication.

Name of Medication	Classification	Action	Dosage	Frequency	Route

- Click on **Return to Room 304**.
- Click on **Medication Room**.
- Prepare the medication you identified in question 8.
- When you have finished the steps of the Preparation Wizard, click on **Return to Medication Room** and then on **304** to go to Stephanie's room.
- Administer the medication, using the five rights of medication administration. After you have collected the appropriate assessment data and are ready for administration, click **Patient Care** and then **Medication Administration**. Verify that the correct patient and medication(s) appear in the left-hand window. Then click the down arrow next to Select. From the drop-down menu, select **Administer** and complete the Administration Wizard by providing any information requested. When the Wizard stops asking for information, click **Administer to Patient**. Specify **Yes** when asked whether this administration should be recorded in the MAR. Finally, click **Finish**.

10. In the mock MAR form below, document the medication you just administered to Stephanie. Indicate the time you gave it in the correct column.

Medication/Dose	2300-0700	0700-1500	1500-2300

Now let's see how you did!

- Click on **Leave the Floor** at the bottom of your screen. From the Floor Menu, select **Look at Your Preceptor's Evaluation**. Then click on **Medication Scorecard**.
- Review the scorecard to see whether or not you correctly administered the appropriate medication. If not, why do you think you were incorrect? According to Table C in this scorecard, what resources should be used and what important assessments should be completed before administering the medication(s)? Did you utilize these resources and perform these assessments correctly?
- Bring a copy of the Medication Scorecard for your instructor to evaluate.

 In your textbook, review Box 21-2 and the Evaluate Behavioral and Physiologic Changes section of Chapter 21.

- Click on **Return to Evaluations** and then **Return to Menu**.
- Click on **Restart the Program** and sign in for Period of Care 2.
- From the Patient List, select Stephanie Brown (Room 304).
- Click on **Go to Nurses' Station**.
- Click on **EPR** and then on **Login**.
- Select **304** as the Patient and **Vital Signs** as the Category.

11. Compare Stephanie's blood pressure and pain scale rating on Wednesday 0700 with her BP and pain rating on Wednesday at 1100.

12. a. Using the FACES pain rating scale below, which face matches Stephanie's description of her headache recorded on Wednesday at 1100?

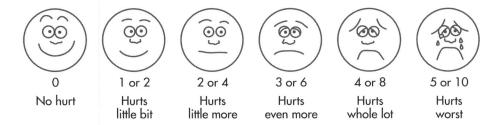

0	1 or 2	2 or 4	3 or 6	4 or 8	5 or 10
No hurt	Hurts little bit	Hurts little more	Hurts even more	Hurts whole lot	Hurts worst

   b. Identify the three scales used in the FACES system.

➡ • Click on **Exit EPR**.
   • Click on **Chart** and then on **304**.
   • Once again, review the **Physician's Orders** for Stephanie.

13. What is ordered that can be administered to alleviate Stephanie's headache?

➡ • Click on **Return to Nurses' Station**.
   • Now click on the **Drug** icon in the lower left corner of your screen.

14. Using the Drug Guide as your reference, complete the following table for the medication you identified in question 13.

Name of Medication	Classification	Action	Dosage	Frequency	Route

• Click on **Return to Nurses' Station**.
• Click on **Chart** and then on **304**.
• Review the **Nurse's Notes** for Tuesday at 2300 and Wednesday at 0600.

15. Based on your assessment of Stephanie at this time, what route would be appropriate for administering the medication you identified in question 13? State your rationale for choosing this route.

 16. Briefly describe the indication(s) for administering baclofen to the child with cerebral palsy. (*Hint:* Use the Drug Guide and see Chapter 32 in your textbook.)

 • Still in the chart, click on **Consultations** and review the Audiology Consult.
• Click on **Return to Nurses' Station** and then **304**.
• Click on **Patient Care** and then on **Nurse–Client Interactions**.
• Select and view the video titled **1145: Teaching—Disease Sequelae**. (*Note:* Check the virtual clock to see whether enough time has elapsed. You can use the fast-forward feature to advance the time by 2-minute intervals if the video is not yet available. Then click again on **Patient Care** and **Nurse-Client Interactions** to refresh the screen.)

 17. Explain the basis for obtaining the audiogram for Stephanie. State the results of the audiogram. (*Hint:* See Table 6-9 and Auditory Testing in Chapter 6 of your textbook.)

Nursing Care of the Hospitalized Child with Cerebral Palsy

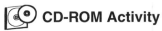 **Reading Assignment:** Family-Centered Care of the Child During Illness and
Hospitalization (Chapter 21): Pain Management; Stressors of
Hospitalization and Children's Reactions; Minimizing Loss of
Control
The Child with Neuromuscular or Muscular Dysfunction
(Chapter 32): Cerebral Palsy; Therapeutic Management

Patient: Stephanie Brown, Room 304

Objectives:

1. Discuss the special needs of a child with cerebral palsy.
2. Describe the issues involved in discharge planning and home care of the child with cerebral palsy.
3. Identify measures to decrease anxiety in a child and family with meningitis.

Exercise 1

 CD-ROM Activity

50 minutes

- Sign in to work at Pacific View Regional Hospital for Period of Care 3. (*Note:* If you are already in the virtual hospital from a previous exercise, click on **Leave the Floor** and then **Restart the Program** to get to the sign-in window.)
- From the Patient List, select Stephanie Brown (Room 304).
- Click on **Go to Nurses' Station**.
- Click on **304** to go to the patient's room.
- Click on **Patient Care** and then **Nurse-Client Interactions**.
- Select and view the video titled **1500: Assessment—IV Site**. (*Note:* Check the virtual clock to see whether enough time has elapsed. You can use the fast-forward feature to advance the time by 2-minute intervals if the video is not yet available. Then click again on **Patient Care** and **Nurse-Client Interactions** to refresh the screen.)

1. How did the nurse describe the IV site in the video? What are the implications of her findings?

- Click on **Patient Care** and then **Nurse-Client Interactions**.
- Now select and view the video titled **1510: Nurse-Patient Communication**. (*Note:* Check the virtual clock to see whether enough time has elapsed. You can use the fast-forward feature to advance the time by 2-minute intervals if the video is not yet available. Then click again on **Patient Care** and **Nurse-Client Interactions** to refresh the screen.)

2. The nurse in the video states that she will apply EMLA cream before restarting Stephanie's IV. What is the purpose of doing this?

Let's take a virtual leap in time to see whether the EMLA cream was actually applied.

- First, click on **Leave the Floor** and then **Restart the Program**.
- Sign in to work with Stephanie Brown for Period of Care 4.
- Click on **MAR** and then on tab **304**. (*Remember:* You are not able to visit patients or administer medications during Period of Care 4. You are able to review patient records only.)
- Review Stephanie's MAR for Wednesday at 1900.

3. At what time was the EMLA cream administered? Why should the nurse wait 60 minutes after EMLA is applied to the skin before the IV is restarted?

Now, let's return to Period of Care 3 to continue your care for Stephanie Brown.

- Once again, click on **Leave the Floor** and then **Restart the Program**.
- Sign in to work with Stephanie Brown for Period of Care 3.
- Click on **Go to Nurses' Station**.
- Click on **Chart** and then on **304**.
- Click on **History and Physical** and review.
- Click on **Nursing Admissions** and review.

4. List the predisposing maternal and perinatal factors in Stephanie's history that may have contributed to the development of cerebral palsy (CP).

➡ • Click on **Consultations** and read the PT/OT consult.

5. State the findings of the PT/OT consult.

6. What specific therapy is recommended for Stephanie by the physical therapist based on the findings during the consult?

7. What is an ankle-foot orthosis (AFO)? When did Stephanie start wearing an AFO? State the purpose of her AFO. (*Hint:* See Therapeutic Management of Cerebral Palsy in Chapter 32 of your textbook.)

➡ • Click on **Nurse's Notes**.
• Review the Nurse's Notes from the ED admission through Wednesday.

8. What specific request does Stephanie's mother make of the social worker? (*Hint:* Read the note on Tuesday at 1500.)

9. Describe activities that can help Stephanie's mother cope with the anxiety associated with her daughter's hospitalization and life-threatening illness.

10. Describe age-appropriate activities that can help Stephanie cope with the anxiety associated with hospitalization and respiratory isolation.

 11. What recommendations could you give Stephanie's mother to promote Stephanie's daily bowel movement? (*Hint:* See Constipation in Chapter 24 of your textbook.)

 • Click on **Return to Nurses' Station**.
• Click on **304** to go to Stephanie's room.
• Click on **Patient Care** and then on **Nurse-Client Interactions**.
• Select and view the video titled **1530: Preventive Measures**. (*Note:* Check the virtual clock to see whether enough time has elapsed. You can use the fast-forward feature to advance the time by 2-minute intervals if the video is not yet available. Then click again on **Patient Care** and **Nurse-Client Interactions** to refresh the screen.)

12. What specific recommendation does the physical therapist make to Stephanie's mother on the consult note and during the video?

LESSON 16

Care of the Infant with Respiratory Distress

 Reading Assignment: Communication and Physical Assessment of the Child
(Chapter 6): Lungs
Pediatric Variations of Nursing Interventions (Chapter 22):
Oxygen Therapy; Aerosol Therapy; Medication—Oral
Administration
The Child with Respiratory Dysfunction (Chapter 23):
Respiratory Syncytial Virus and Bronchiolitis
The Child with Gastrointestinal Dysfunction (Chapter 24):
Water Balance in Infants
Vital Signs (Inside back cover of textbook)

Patient: Carrie Richards, Room 303

Objectives:

1. Recognize signs of acute respiratory distress in an infant.
2. Describe interventions to treat respiratory distress in an infant.
3. Describe the nursing care of an infant with RSV/bronchiolitis.

Exercise 1

 Writing Activity

30 minutes

1. What is RSV? Briefly describe the characteristic progression of this illness in children.
Also identify any associated clinical manifestations.

2. How is this illness transmitted?

3. What steps can be taken to reduce or prevent the transmission of this illness?

4. What medication may be given as prophylactic treatment for RSV in high-risk patients? Who should receive the medication, and when should this medication be administered? How is the medication given?

Exercise 2

 CD-ROM Activity

 50 minutes

- Sign in to work at Pacific View Regional Hospital for Period of Care 1. (*Note:* If you are already in the virtual hospital from a previous exercise, click on **Leave the Floor** and then **Restart the Program** to get to the sign-in window.)
- From the Patient List, select Carrie Richards (Room 303).
- Click on **Go to Nurses' Station**.
- Click on **Chart** and then on **303** for Carrie's chart.
- Click on **Emergency Department** and review this record.

1. What are Carrie's vital signs on admission to the ED at 1630? Put an asterisk next to any findings that are out of normal range for a child her age.

2. Briefly describe the findings for Carrie recorded in the ED Systems Review and in the ED Nurse's Note at 1800. Put an asterisk next to any findings that are abnormal for a child Carrie's age.

3. List the five cardinal clinical signs of respiratory distress (RD) in an infant.

➤ • Still in the Emergency Department section of the chart, compare the findings in the ED Nurse's Notes at 1800 and 1900.

4. What clinical signs documented by the nurse indicate a change in Carrie's respiratory status at 1900?

5. What specific intervention is performed to improve Carrie's oxygenation status?

6. What medication is administered to Carrie to improve her respiratory status in the ED?

7. Describe the intended effect of this medication in a child with bronchiolitis/RSV who is wheezing and has a lower airway infection. (*Hint:* See Asthma: Drug Therapy in Chapter 23 of your textbook.)

8. Describe how this medication is administered in an infant Carrie's age. What is the rationale for this method of administration?

9. List two side effects of this medication.

10. Identify priority assessments that need to be performed after the nebulizer treatment is given.

11. What is the primary medical diagnosis listed for Carrie?

12. List two nursing diagnoses for Carrie based on your review of her status in the ED.

13. In the 1800 ED nurse's notes, an important clue is given in relation to the severity of Carrie's status. What might lead you to conclude that her condition is poor? (*Hint:* Consider her age and developmental status.)

➤ • Still in Carrie's chart, click on **Laboratory Reports**.

14. Below, fill in Carrie's laboratory values recorded in the ED at 1800 on Tuesday.

Chemistry	Results	Arterial Blood Gas	Results
Glucose		pH	
Sodium (serum)		PaO_2	
Potassium		$PaCO_2$	
Chloride		Oxygen sat	
CO_2			
Creatinine			
BUN			
Calcium			

Urinalysis	Results	Hematology	Results
Color		WBC	
Clarity		RBC	
Glucose		Hgb	
Bilirubin		Hct	
Blood		Platelets	
Spec gravity		Differential	
pH		Segs	
Protein		Bands	
Ketones		Lymphocytes	
WBC		Monocytes	
		Eosinophils	
		Basophils	

 15. Which lab values in the table in question 14 are out of normal range for a child Carrie's age? (*Hint:* See Appendix C in your textbook.)

→ • Click on **Emergency Department**. Once again, review the ED nurse's notes for 1900 on Tuesday.

16. How is Carrie's respiratory status described? What interventions other than the nebulized medication administration and oxygen were performed to improve Carrie's respiratory status? State the rationale for the intervention performed.

 17. List the clinical signs, physical assessment findings, and any laboratory values that provide a basis for determining Carrie's hydration status on admission to the ED. (*Hint:* Refer to Dehydration in Chapter 24 and Parenteral Fluid Therapy in Chapter 22 of your textbook.)

18. Describe the intervention(s) used to hydrate Carrie in the ED.

19. List two reasons Carrie is *not* a candidate for oral hydration in the ED.

20. Describe important assessment data that should be documented regarding Carrie's IV site.

17

Care of the Hospitalized Infant

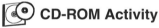 **Reading Assignment:** Communication and Physical Assessment of the Child
(Chapter 6): Lungs
Pediatric Variations of Nursing Interventions (Chapter 22):
Controlling Elevated Temperatures
The Child with Respiratory Dysfunction (Chapter 23):
Respiratory Syncytial Virus and Bronchiolitis

Patient: Carrie Richards, Room 303

Objectives:

1. Identify physical assessment of the infant with respiratory distress.
2. Describe the nursing care of an infant with RSV/bronchiolitis.

Exercise 1

 CD-ROM Activity

20 minutes

- Sign in to work at Pacific View Regional Hospital for Period of Care 1. (*Note:* If you are
  already in the virtual hospital from a previous exercise, click on **Leave the Floor** and then
  Restart the Program to get to the sign-in window.)
- From the Patient List, select Carrie Richards (Room 303).
- Click on **Get Report**.
- Click on **Go to Nurses' Station**.
- Click **Chart** and then on **303**.
- Click on and review the **Emergency Department** records.
- Click on and review **History and Physical**.
- Click on and review the **Nursing Admission** and the **Physician's Orders** for Tuesday 1700
  and 2300.

1. Briefly summarize Carrie's health history since birth.

2. Is Carrie's immunization status current? If not, list the immunization(s) she should receive as soon as possible. (*Hint:* See Childhood Immunizations in Chapter 10 of your textbook.)

• Before leaving the chart, record Carrie's physical assessment findings on admission in the middle column of the table in question 3. (*Hint:* You can find these in the Emergency Department record.)
• After recording these findings, click on **Return to Nurses' Station**.
• Click on **303** to go to Carrie's room.
• Click on **Patient Care** and then **Physical Assessment**.
• Perform a focused assessment by selecting the various body areas and system subcategories as needed to complete question 3.

3. Record your findings from the physical assessment (her current in-room findings) in the far-right column below. Then compare these current findings with those obtained on admission to the ED (those you found in her chart).

Findings	Admission 1700 Tuesday	Current Findings
Respiratory effort		
Breath sounds		
Adventitious lung sounds		
Sensory/activity level		
Capillary refill		
Pulses		
Supplemental oxygen		

• Still in Carrie's room, click on **Patient Care** and then **Nurse-Client Interactions**.

• Select and view the video titled **0730: Patient Assessment**. (*Note:* Check the virtual clock to see whether enough time has elapsed. You can use the fast-forward feature to advance the time by 2-minute intervals if the video is not yet available. Then click again on **Patient Care** and **Nurse-Client Interactions** to refresh the screen.)

4. How does the nurse assess Carrie's respiratory status in the video?

5. Carrie is 3½ months old. At this age, breathing is primarily:

   a. abdominal.
   b. diaphragmatic.

 • Click on **Take Vital Signs**.

6. Record Carrie's vital sign results below.

   T

   HR

   RR

   O$_2$ sat

   BP

7. Based on Carrie's current physical assessment findings and vital signs, what conclusion might be drawn about her respiratory status and general health at this time?

• Click on **EPR** and **Login**.

• Select **303** from the Patient drop-down menu.

• Choose various categories as needed to record the vital signs and physical assessment finding you gathered in Carrie's room. Be sure to include respiratory findings and IV status. (*Note:* The EPR may be printed for instructor evaluation.)

Exercise 2

 CD-ROM Activity

 45 minutes

- Sign in to work at Pacific View Regional Hospital for Period of Care 3. (*Note:* If you are already in the virtual hospital from a previous exercise, click on **Leave the Floor** and then **Restart the Program** to get to the sign-in window.)
- From the Patient List, select Carrie Richards (Room 303).
- Click on **Go to Nurses' Station**.
- Click on **Chart** and then on **303**.
- Review the **Nurse's Notes**.
- Click on **Return to Nurses' Station**.
- Click on **EPR** and then **Login**.
- Select **303** as the Patient and **Respiratory** as the Category.

1. Summarize Carrie's respiratory status at 1300 on Wednesday based on the 1240 nurse's notes and 1215 respiratory assessment data in the EPR.

 • Still in the EPR, change the category to **Vital Signs**.

2. What is Carrie's body temperature at 1445?

➡ • Click on **Exit EPR**.
- Click on **MAR** and then on tab **303**.

3. What medication does Carrie have ordered for fever or irritability?

Now let's go to the Medication Room and prepare to administer all of the 1500 medications ordered for Carrie.

➡ • First, click on **Return to Nurses' Station**.
- Next, click on **Medication Room**.
- Click on **MAR** to determine what medications Carrie should receive for 1500. You may review the MAR at any time to verify the correct medication order. (*Hint:* Remember to look at the patient name on the MAR to make sure you have the correct record—you must click on

the tab with Carrie's room number within the MAR.) Click on **Return to Medication Room** after reviewing the correct MAR.

- Click on **Unit Dosage** and then on drawer **303**.

- Select the medications you would like to administer. For each medication you select, click on **Put Medication on Tray**. When you are finished, click on **Close Drawer**.

- Click **View Medication Room**.

- Now click on **Automated System** and **Login**.

- Select the correct patient and drawer according to the medication you want to administer. (*Hint:* This automated system is for controlled substances only.) Then click **Open Drawer**.

- Select the medication you would like to administer, click on **Put Medication on Tray**, and then click **Close Drawer**.

- Click **View Medication Room**.

- Click on **Preparation** and select the medication to administer.

- Click **Prepare** and wait for the Preparation Wizard to appear. If the Wizard requests information, provide your answer(s), and then click **Next**.

- Choose the correct patient and then click **Finish**.

- Repeat the previous three steps until all medications that you want to administer are prepared.

- You can click on **Review Your Medications** and then click **Return to Medication Room** when ready. Once you are back in the Medication Room, go directly to Carrie's room by clicking on **303** at the bottom of the screen.

- In Carrie's room, administer the medications, using the five rights of medication administration. After you have collected the appropriate assessment data and are ready for administration, click **Patient Care** and then **Medication Administration**. Verify that the correct patient and medication(s) appear in the left-hand window. Then click the down arrow next to Select. From the drop-down menu, select **Administer** and complete the Administration Wizard by providing any information requested. When the Wizard stops asking for information, click **Administer to Patient**. Specify **Yes** when asked whether this administration should be recorded in the MAR. Finally, click **Finish**. Complete these steps for each medication you wish to administer.

Now let's see how you did!

- Click on **Leave the Floor** at the bottom of your screen. From the Floor Menu, select **Look at Your Preceptor's Evaluation**. Then click on **Medication Scorecard**.

- Review the scorecard to see whether or not you correctly administered the appropriate medication(s). If not, why do you think you were incorrect? According to Table C in this scorecard, what resources should be used and what important assessments should be completed before administering the medication(s)? Did you use these resources and perform these assessments correctly?

- Print a copy of the Medication Scorecard for your instructor to evaluate.

   4. How does the nurse evaluate pain or discomfort in an infant Carrie's age? (*Hint:* See Pain Assessment in Chapter 21 of your textbook.)

• Click on **Return to Evaluations** and then **Return to Menu**.
• Click on **Restart the Program** and sign in for Period of Care 3.
• From the Patient List, select Carrie Richards (Room 303).
• Click on **Go to Nurses' Station** and then **303**.
• Click on **Patient Care** and then **Nurse-Client Interactions**.
• Select and view the video titled **1500: Teaching—Oral Medication**. (*Note:* Check the virtual clock to see whether enough time has elapsed. You can use the fast-forward feature to advance the time by 2-minute intervals if the video is not yet available. Then click again on **Patient Care** and **Nurse-Client Interactions** to refresh the screen.)

5. How does the nurse teach Carrie's mother (Brenda) to administer Carrie's oral medication?

6. What statement(s) does Brenda make about Carrie's eating habits in the last few days before admission?

7. What interrelated factors should the nurse consider when an infant has a compromising respiratory illness such as RSV/bronchiolitis and the infant's food intake is decreased?

 8. What are the implications of these findings for an infant in relation to hydration status and present illness? (*Hint:* See Water Balance in Infants in Chapter 24 of your textbook.)

9. What concerns does Carrie's mother express about her daughter's nutritional status?

10. How does the nurse address Brenda's concerns about Carrie's nutritional status?

11. An infant's illness and hospitalization may represent a significant stressor for a single mother and her infant. What can the nursing staff do to minimize Brenda's anxiety about her child's hospitalization? (*Hint:* See Preventing or Minimizing Separation in Chapter 21 of your textbook.)

Nutritional Assessment and Discharge Planning

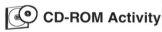 **Reading Assignment:** Health Problems of Infants (Chapter 11): Growth Failure
Family-Centered Care of the Child During Illness and Hospital-
ization (Chapter 21): Infants; Nursing Care of the Family;
Discharge Assessment

Patient: Carrie Richards, Room 303

Objectives:

1. Assess the nutritional status of the infant with suspected growth failure.
2. Describe the nursing care of the infant with growth failure, including family interventions
   for home care and management.

Exercise 1

 CD-ROM Activity

20 minutes

- Sign in to work at Pacific View Regional Hospital for Period of Care 1. (*Note:* If you are
  already in the virtual hospital from a previous exercise, click on **Leave the Floor** and then
  Restart the Program to get to the sign-in window.)
- From the Patient List, select Carrie Richards (Room 303).
- Click on **Get Report**.
- Click on **Go to Nurses' Station**.
- Click on **Chart** and then on **303**.
- Click on and review the **Emergency Department** and the **History and Physical**.
- Click on and review the **Nursing Admission** and the **Physician's Notes** for Tuesday at 1700
  and 2300.

1. What was Carrie's weight on admission to the ED?

2. What observations were made regarding the appearance of Carrie's body size in the ED?

3. What additional observations were made by the staff that address Carrie's overall nutritional status?

4. What is Carrie's secondary medical diagnosis in the ED?

5. What is the rationale for weighing Carrie again on Wednesday morning at 0755?

6. Review the CDC growth chart on the following page (Birth to 36 months: Girls—Length-for-Age and Weight-for-Age Percentiles). Plot Carrie's admission weight and length on the chart.

    Carrie is just below the _____ percentile for weight-for-age and at the _____ percentile for length-for-age at 3½ months.

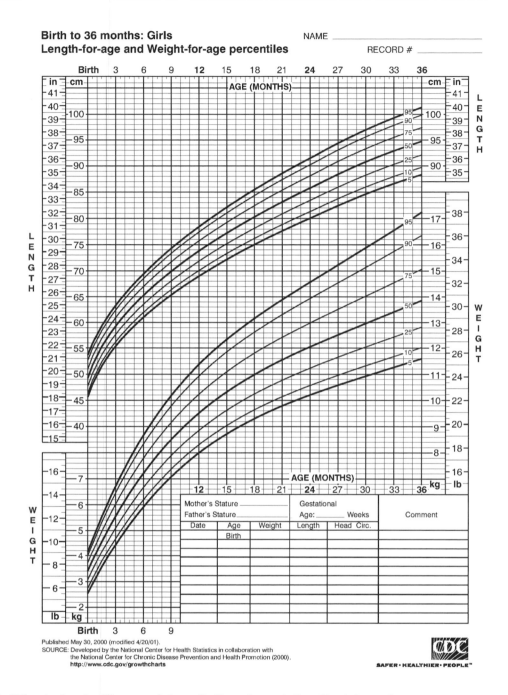

Birth to 36 months: Girls
Length-for-age and Weight-for-age percentiles

NAME _____

RECORD # _____

Published May 30, 2000 (modified 4/20/01).
SOURCE: Developed by the National Center for Health Statistics in collaboration with
the National Center for Chronic Disease Prevention and Health Promotion (2000).
http://www.cdc.gov/growthcharts

7. What is the significance of these findings for an infant Carrie's age?

➤ • Once again, review Carrie's **History and Physical** and **Nursing Admission** in the chart.

8. In the dietary history there is significant information regarding Carrie's feedings. What does the mother say she has been feeding her daughter? (Include amounts and frequency as applicable.)

 9. What is the significance of this information? (*Hint:* See Nutrition, The First Six Months, in Chapter 10 in your textbook.)

10. What is the rationale for the addition of rice cereal to a nighttime bottle?

11. Is the practice of putting an infant to sleep with a nighttime bottle recommended? Why?

> * Click on **Return to Nurses' Station**.
> * Click on **303** to go to Carrie's room.
> * Click on **Patient Care** and then on **Nurse-Client Interactions**.
> * Select and view the video titled **0800: Assessment—Fact Finding**. (*Note:* Check the virtual clock to see whether enough time has elapsed. You can use the fast-forward feature to advance the time by 2-minute intervals if the video is not yet available. Then click again on **Patient Care** and **Nurse-Client Interactions** to refresh the screen.)

12. What assessment does the nurse in the video tell the mother she will make to assess Carrie's ability to tolerate feedings in relation to her condition?

13. What additional observations might the nurse make at the time of feeding?

 14. How is the diagnosis of growth failure established? (*Hint:* See Growth Failure, Diagnostic Evaluation, in Chapter 11 in your textbook.)

Exercise 2

 CD-ROM Activity

 15 minutes

- Sign in to work at Pacific View Regional Hospital for Period of Care 2. (*Note:* If you are already in the virtual hospital from a previous exercise, click on **Leave the Floor** and then **Restart the Program** to get to the sign-in window.)
- From the Patient List, select Carrie Richards (Room 303).
- Click on **Go to Nurses' Station**.
- Click on **Chart** and then **303**.
- Click on **Consultations** and read the Dietary/Nutrition Consult.

1. What does the dietitian report regarding Carrie's nutritional status?

2. According to the consult findings, what additional information is discovered about how Carrie is fed that has a significant impact on the number of calories she has been receiving?

3. How might the nurse assess the report that Carrie spits up frequently after feedings?

→ • Click on **Chart** and then on **303**.
 • Click on **Consultations**.
 • In the Dietary Consult, review the dietitian's plan for Carrie to achieve catch-up growth in the next few weeks.
 • Now click on **Nurse's Notes** and review the notes for Wednesday at 1240, 1425, and 1500.

4. Briefly summarize Carrie's feeding pattern since the acute phase of respiratory distress has resolved and her breathing has improved.

5. What is MCT oil? Why is it added to Carrie's formula?

6. Write two measurable outcomes for weight gain and caloric (formula) intake for Carrie for the next few days. Include specifics on how these outcomes will be measured.

7. Some interventions have been addressed dealing with Carrie's growth failure. Identify additional nursing interventions that would be appropriate to implement in the hospital setting to help the mother care for Carrie.

Exercise 3

 CD-ROM Activity

 10 minutes

- Sign in to work at Pacific View Regional Hospital for Period of Care 3. (*Note:* If you are already in the virtual hospital from a previous exercise, click on **Leave the Floor** and then **Restart the Program** to get to the sign-in window.)
- From the Patient List, select Carrie Richards (Room 303).
- Click on **Go to Nurses' Station**.
- Click on **Chart** and then on **303**.
- Click on **Consultations** and review the Social Service Consult at 1430 on Wednesday.
- While in the chart, also review the **Nursing Admission** and the **History and Physical**.

1. Describe Carrie's mother's family situation, marital status, sources of economic support, and any other factors that may influence her ability to care for herself and her daughter.

2. Devise a plan for post-discharge follow-up for Carrie and her mother. Consider the mother's lack of transportation, the need for close medical follow-up to assess Carrie's progress over the next few weeks, and the limited family resources. Set up the plan for Carrie's discharge on Thursday morning and evaluate the feasibility of the plan, assuming that her respiratory status continues to improve as it has since admission Tuesday evening.

George Gonzalez

LESSON — **19** —

Emergent Care of the Child with Diabetic Ketoacidosis

Reading Assignment: Health Promotion of the School-Age Child and Family (Chapter 15)

Family-Centered Care of the Child During Illness and Hospitalization (Chapter 21): School-Age Children

The Child with Gastrointestinal Dysfunction (Chapter 24): Dehydration

The Child with Endocrine Dysfunction (Chapter 29): Diabetes Mellitus

Patient: George Gonzalez, Room 301

Objectives:

1. Recognize the clinical manifestations of diabetic ketoacidosis (DKA) in a child with type 1 diabetes mellitus.
2. Describe the pathophysiology of DKA in a child with type 1 diabetes mellitus.
3. Describe the nursing care of the child with DKA.
4. Identify significant diagnostic laboratory tests in the management of type 1 diabetes mellitus.

Exercise 1

 CD-ROM Activity

 30 minutes

- Sign in to work at Pacific View Regional Hospital for Period of Care 1. (*Note:* If you are already in the virtual hospital from a previous exercise, click on **Leave the Floor** and then **Restart the Program** to get to the sign-in window.)
- From the Patient List, select George Gonzalez (Room 301).
- Click on **Go to Nurses' Station**.
- Click on **Chart** and then on **301** for George's record.
- Click on **Emergency Department**.

141

1. What were George's primary and secondary medical diagnoses on admission to the ED?

2. List three clinical manifestations of DKA.

3. What is the significance of vomiting in a child who has DKA?

4. List altered neurologic signs the nurse should be alert for in a child with DKA.

→ • Click on **Laboratory Reports** and review the initial lab work drawn in the ED at 1730 on Tuesday.

5. What was George's blood glucose result on admission?

6. List the normal blood glucose values for a child George's age. (*Hint:* See Appendix C in your textbook.)

7. Complete the table below with George's lab values and normal parameters.

Lab Values	George's Values	Normal Values
Sodium (serum)		
Potassium (serum)		
BUN		
Creatinine		
CO_2		
Urine ketones		
Urine glucose		
Urine specific gravity		
Arterial pH		
$PaCO_2$		
PaO_2		
WBC		
Hgb		
Hct		
Platelets		
RBC		

8. Based on George's lab values in questions 5 and 7, is the diagnosis of DKA supported at this time?

9. Identify the initial intervention performed in the ED to rehydrate George.

10. What nursing observations are particularly important for a child with DKA who is receiving intravenous fluids? (*Hint:* See Management of DKA in Chapter 29 in your textbook.)

11. What is the significance of monitoring cardiac function in a child with DKA?

→ • Click on **Physician's Orders** and review the orders for George in the ED at 1730.

12. What medication is ordered?

To answer the following questions, refer to the Diabetes Mellitus in Chapter 29 in your textbook.

13. What is the preferred method for administering insulin to a patient with DKA?

14. How is George's insulin administered in the ED at 1730?

15. What is the significance of admitting the child with DKA to an intensive care unit?

16. What are Kussmaul respirations?

17. What is the significance of Kussmaul respirations in ketoacidosis?

Care of the Hospitalized Child with Type 1 Diabetes Mellitus

——————————————————————————————————

 Reading Assignment: The Child with Endocrine Dysfunction (Chapter 29): Diabetes Mellitus

Patient: George Gonzalez, Room 301

Objectives:

1. Differentiate between type 1 and type 2 diabetes mellitus (DM).
2. Differentiate between the types of insulin used in the child with type 1 diabetes mellitus.
3. Identify specific learning and emotional needs of the preadolescent with a chronic illness.

Exercise 1

 CD-ROM Activity

45 minutes

*   Sign in to work at Pacific View Regional Hospital for Period of Care 1. (*Note:* If you are already in the virtual hospital from a previous exercise, click on **Leave the Floor** and then **Restart the Program** to get to the sign-in window.)
*   From the Patient List, select George Gonzalez (Room 301).
*   Click on **Go to Nurses' Station**.
*   Click on **Chart** and then on **301** for George's record.
*   Click on and review the **History and Physical** and **Nursing Admission** sections of the chart.

1. List the three Ps that are cardinal signs associated with type 1 diabetes mellitus. Briefly explain the significance of each term.

2. In the table below, identify the main differences between type 1 and type 2 diabetes mellitus.

Characteristics	Type 1 DM	Type 2 DM
Type of onset		
Sex ratio		
Presenting symptoms		
Nutritional status		
Serum insulin (natural)		
Chronic complications		
Ketoacidosis		
Therapy Used		
Insulin		
Oral agents		
Diet only		

3. The signs and symptoms of diabetes mellitus (DM) may mimic those of other illnesses and may be overlooked. What are some of the illnesses with similar signs and symptoms that may cause one to overlook DM?

4. What was George's HgbA1C (glycosylated hemoglobin) on admission to the ED?

5. The primary goals of DM treatment are to maintain glucose levels of _____ mg/dL

and a glycosylated hemoglobin (HgbA1C) less than _____%.

6. What is the significance of the HgbA1C in a person with diabetes mellitus in relation to compliance and long-term complications?

• Click on **Return to Nurses' Station** and then on **301**.
   • Click on **Patient Care** and then **Nurse-Client Interactions**.
   • Select and view the video titled **0730: Supervision—Glucose Testing**. (*Note:* Check the virtual clock to see whether enough time has elapsed. You can use the fast-forward feature to advance the time by 2-minute intervals if the video is not yet available. Then click again on **Patient Care** and **Nurse-Client Interactions** to refresh the screen.)

7. What does George say about checking his glucose at home?

8. What skill does the nurse ask George to perform during this interaction?

9. What is the significance of the nurse observing George check his glucose instead of checking it for him?

10. What was George's fingerstick blood glucose at 0745 on Wednesday?

 • Click on **Chart** and then on **301**.
   • Click on **Physician's Orders** and review the orders written at 2200 on Tuesday.
   • Click on **Return to Room 301**.
   • Now click on **MAR** and review George's MAR for Wednesday morning.

11. What intervention should occur once George has checked his blood glucose level before breakfast?

12. In addition to monitoring his glucose levels, what additional psychomotor skill should George be expected to perform in relation to diabetic management?

13. List the doses and types of insulin George is to administer before his breakfast.

14. What step should be taken to prevent hypoglycemia when a rapid-acting insulin is administered?

Insulin is now available in a number of premixed forms that make administration easier. These forms include the insulin pump and insulin pen. The insulin pump and pen may not be available to all children because of cost and skill level. George may be a candidate for administering insulin with an insulin pen.

15. Briefly describe the advantages of an insulin pen for a person George's age.

16. What is the rationale for using both types of insulin throughout the day?

17. Briefly describe how you would draw up the following: lispro 6 units and NPH 12 units. Be specific about the order in which you would complete these steps. (*Remember:* Clear insulin, then cloudy insulin.)

18. Match each type of insulin with its corresponding description. Each description may match more than one type of insulin.

Type of Insulin	Description
_____ Humalog (lispro H) NovoLog (aspart)	a. Rapid-acting insulin
_____ NPH or Lente	b. Intermediate-acting insulin
_____ Regular	c. Long-acting insulin
_____ UltraLente	d. Injected immediately before meals
_____ Lantus (glargine)	

➤ • Click on **Return to Room 301**.
  • Click on **Patient Care** and then on **Nurse-Client Interactions**.
  • Select and view the video titled **0745: Self-Administering Insulin**. (*Note:* Check the virtual clock to see whether enough time has elapsed. You can use the fast-forward feature to advance the time by 2-minute intervals if the video is not yet available. Then click again on **Patient Care** and **Nurse-Client Interactions** to refresh the screen.)

19. In the video, what specific task does the nurse ask George to perform?

20. In this video interaction, how does the nurse evaluate George's understanding of his diabetes?

21. Based on your observation of George's actions in this video and his responses to the nurse about his condition, what conclusions would you draw about George's knowledge regarding diabetes and his subsequent ability to perform glucose monitoring and insulin injection?

22. In the interactions with the nurse, George makes a statement about how he has managed his diabetes previously. What does he say about his daily monitoring of glucose and administration of insulin before going to school?

21

Diabetes Care and Self-Management

/👓 Reading Assignment: Health Promotion of the School-Age Child and Family (Chapter 15): Nutrition

Family-Centered Care of the Child During Illness and Hospitalization (Chapter 21): School-Age Children; Discharge Assessment

The Child with Endocrine Dysfunction (Chapter 29): Diabetes Mellitus

Patient: George Gonzalez, Room 301

Objectives:

1. Describe the significance of glucose monitoring, diet, and exercise in the management of the child with type 1 diabetes mellitus.
2. Discuss the impact of a chronic illness on the preadolescent child and family.
3. Identify potential complications of type 1 diabetes in relation to poor glycemic control.
4. Identify specific learning needs of the preadolescent with a chronic illness.

Exercise 1

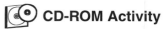 **CD-ROM Activity**

 55 minutes

- Sign in to work at Pacific View Regional Hospital for Period of Care 2. (*Note:* If you are already in the virtual hospital from a previous exercise, click on **Leave the Floor** and then **Restart the Program** to get to the sign-in window.)
- From the Patient List, select George Gonzalez (Room 301).
- Click on **Go to Nurses' Station**.
- Click on **Chart** and then on **301** for George Gonzalez's record.
- Click on and review the **Nurse's Notes** and **Physician's Notes**.
- Click on **Return to Nurses' Station** and then on **301** to go to George's room.
- Click on **Patient Care** and then on **Nurse-Client Interactions**.

- Select and view the video titled **1115: Teaching—Disease Process**. (*Note:* Check the virtual clock to see whether enough time has elapsed. You can use the fast-forward feature to advance the time by 2-minute intervals if the video is not yet available. Then click again on **Patient Care** and **Nurse-Client Interactions** to refresh the screen.)
- Now view the video titled **1130: Teaching—Managing Symptoms**.

1. What does George's mother say about his diabetes management?

2. What does George's mother tell the nurse about recognizing George's need for insulin?

3. The nurse discusses with the mother signs indicating George may need insulin. What are the signs of hyperglycemia in a child George's age?

4. During these two video sessions, what is the nurse evaluating in regard to knowledge of diabetes management?

5. What does George tell the nurse about the signs of hypoglycemia? What does he think he should do if he feels hypoglycemic?

➡ • *Note:* To answer the following two questions you may need to return to Period of Care 1 and view the nurse's interactions with George and his mother. If you need help changing periods of care, see page 18 in the **Getting Started** section of this workbook.

6. Briefly summarize your impressions regarding the following issues.

   a. George's previous management of diabetes in relation to glucose monitoring and insulin administration:

   b. George's mother's knowledge about the importance of daily diabetes management:

7. Briefly summarize the main teaching points the nurse has covered up to this point with George and his mother regarding diabetes management.

8. What could the nurse emphasize with George and his mother about diabetes management to help control his blood glucose and prevent further hospitalizations?

→ • Click on **Chart** and then on **301**.
  • Review the **History and Physical** and the **Nursing Admission**.
  • Next, click on **Consultations** and review the Psychiatric Consult.

9. According to the History and Physical, George has been hospitalized for problems with diabetes. What specific problems has he had with diabetes management in the last 4 months?

10. List two nursing diagnoses for George based on what you have learned from his chart and the nurse-client video interactions.

11. Briefly describe George's family situation (parents, siblings, primary care provider).

12. There are insights to George's previous diabetes management patterns found in the Nursing Admission, History and Physical, and Psychiatric Consult in the chart. List four factors that contribute to George's noncompliance with the diabetes regimen in the last 4 months.

13. What involvement is expected of George's family, given his age and developmental stage? (*Hint:* See Diabetes Mellitus Family Support in Chapter 29 of your textbook.)

14. George has had diabetes for 4 years. Briefly describe the effect of a chronic illness such as diabetes on a preadolescent and his family. (*Hint:* To learn more about the impact of illness or disability on the preadolescent, see Impact of the Child's Chronic Illness in Chapter 18 in your textbook.)

Exercise 2

 CD-ROM Activity

 20 minutes

- Sign in to work at Pacific View Regional Hospital for Period of Care 3. (*Note:* If you are already in the virtual hospital from a previous exercise, click on **Leave the Floor** and then **Restart the Program** to get to the sign-in window.)
- From the Patient List, select George Gonzalez (Room 301).
- Click on **Go to Nurses' Station**.
- Click on **Chart** and then on **301** for George's record.
- Click on **Consultations** and review the Nutrition Consult.
- Click on **Return to Nurses' Station**.
- Click on **301** to go to George's room.
- Inside his room, click on **Patient Care** and then on **Nurse-Client Interactions**.
- Select and view the video titled **1500: Teaching—Diabetic Diet**. (*Note:* Check the virtual clock to see whether enough time has elapsed. You can use the fast-forward feature to advance the time by 2-minute intervals if the video is not yet available. Then click again on **Patient Care** and **Nurse-Client Interactions** to refresh the screen.)

1. What is George's recommended dietary intake?

2. What does the nurse discuss with George in regard to his food intake?

3. What has been George's pattern of eating in the last several months?

4. Describe the relationship of food intake to insulin injections in a child with type 1 DM.

5. How does carbohydrate (CHO) counting give more flexibility in making food choices and administering insulin in children with type 1 DM?

→ • Click on **Patient Care** and then **Nurse-Client Interactions**.

• Select and view the video titled **1535: Teaching—Effects of Exercise**. (*Note:* Check the virtual clock to see whether enough time has elapsed. You can use the fast-forward feature to advance the time by 2-minute intervals if the video is not yet available. Then click again on **Patient Care** and **Nurse-Client Interactions** to refresh the screen.)

6. What activity does George say he really likes?

7. Why is exercise an important part of the management of type 1 diabetes?

8. Identify important items in the following areas that the nurse should discuss with George in relation to diabetes management and exercise.

 a. Glucose monitoring

b. Carbohydrate intake

c. When not to exercise

d. Signs of activity intolerance

9. What specific intervention does George promise to get involved in following discharge that is aimed at helping him manage his diabetes effectively? (*Hint:* If necessary, return to George's chart and review the **Consultations**.)

Notes:

Notes: